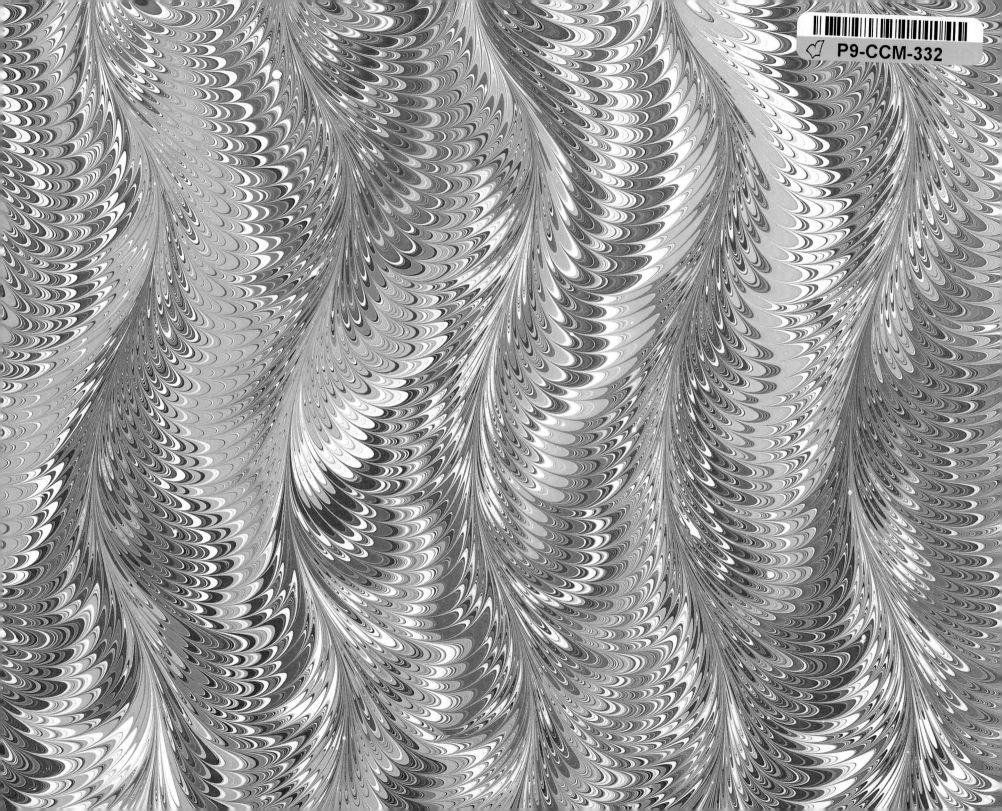

MASKS of the WORLD

Douglas L. Congdon-Martin
and Jim Pieper

In Cooperation with the
California Heritage Museum
Santa Monica, California

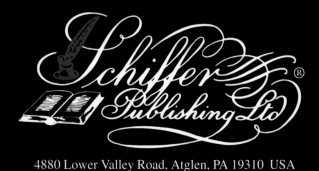

Schiffer Publishing Ltd

4880 Lower Valley Road, Atglen, PA 19310 USA

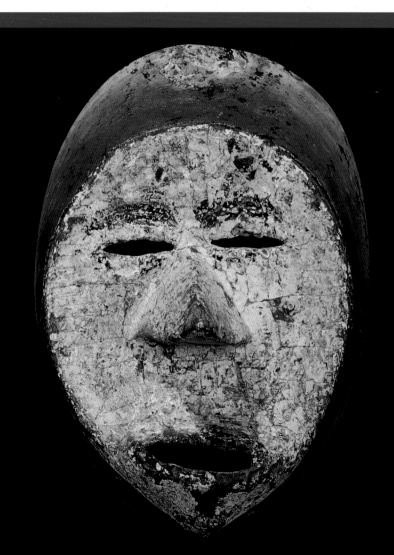

Library of Congress Cataloging-in-Publishing Data
Congdon-Martin, Douglas
Masks of the World / Douglas L. Congdon-Martin and Jim
Pieper ; in cooperation with the California Heritage Museum.
 p. cm.
 Includes bibliographical references.
 ISBN: 0-7643-0968-4 (hardcover)
 1. Masks Exhibitions. 2. Ethnic art Exhibitions. 3. California
Heritage Museum Exhibitions. I. Pieper, Jim. II. California
Heritage Museum. III. Title.
GN419.5.C66   1999
391.4"34--dc21   99-29934
                                                           CIP

Unless otherwise indicated the photos are by Douglas Congdon-
Martin and are copyrighted by Schiffer Publishing Ltd.

Additional copyrighted photos were used with permission from the
following photographers: Jim Pieper, Shirley and David Rowen,
Doran Ross, Lesley Martin. They are credited with their photographs.

Design by Blair Loughrey
Type set in Revue BT/Zurich BT

ISBN: 0-7643-0968-4
Printed in China

Published by Schiffer Publishing Ltd.
4880 Lower Valley Road
Atglen, PA 19310
Phone: (610) 593-1777; Fax: (610) 593-2002
E-mail: Schifferbk@aol.com
Please visit our web site catalog at
www.schifferbooks.com

This book may be purchased from the publisher.
Include $3.95 for shipping.
Please try your bookstore first.
We are interested in hearing from authors
with book ideas on related subjects.
You may write for a free catalog.

In Europe, Schiffer books are distributed by
Bushwood Books
6 Marksbury Rd.
Kew Gardens
Surrey TW9 4JF England
Phone: 44 (0)181 392-8585;
Fax: 44 (0)181 392-9876
E-mail: Bushwd@aol.com

Please try your bookstore first.

We are interested in hearing from authors
with book ideas on related subjects.

CONTENTS

ACKNOWLEDGMENTS

I would like to thank the lenders to the "*Masks of the World*" exhibition for willingly parting with their most precious possessions. I greatly appreciate the time and energy of guest curator and museum Board member Jim Pieper, who visited lenders homes for months on end, and made the difficult final selections of each mask to be displayed in the exhibition. I would also like to acknowledge the efforts of Paul Melzan, who designed the physical wall layout and color scheme of the show, and other staff members at *Pieper and Associates* who worked on the very innovative exhibition labels.

Board member Chase Berke and Buddy Berke co-owners of *Power House/Buddy Berke and Associates* generously provided all of the photography and banner production work displayed in the exhibition. Their support is gratefully appreciated.

I would like to warmly thank staff curator Michael Trotter, who created the installation design, carpenter/preparator Steve Stanley and administrative assistants Stefannie Bernstein and Rudy Vonack for their enthusiastic efforts and hard work on the exhibition. And, most importantly, the exhibition would not be possible without our docent volunteers that keep the doors open by providing informative tours to all that visited the "*Masks of the World*" exhibition.

"*Masks of the World*" is the third California Heritage Museum book published by *Schiffer Publishing, Ltd.* The museum's staff has enjoyed working with Schiffer photographer and co-author Douglas Congdon Martin, and we are grateful to CEO Peter Schiffer and his staff for the opportunity that they have given the museum to share its exhibitions with a far greater audience than those that could personally visit the museum.

Tobi Smith
Executive Director

Lenders to the Exhibition

Amerind Foundation, Inc.
Dr. Richard & Jan Baum
Annette & Seymour Bird
Marlan Clarke
Woods Davy
Helen Epstein, Los Angeles
Joni & Monte Gordon,
    Newspace, Los Angeles
Michael Hamson
Mr. and Mrs. David E. Hayen
Will & Celeste Hughes
Dr. and Mrs. Robert Kuhn
Susan Lerer
Jon and Cari Markell
Ann and Monroe Morgan
Ed Moses
Jim and Jeanne Pieper
Tom & Alma Pirazzini
Larry and Sandy Roseman
Dr. John Ross
Shirley & David Rowen
Mayer and Faith Schames
Jerry Solomon, Los Angeles, CA
Dr. Harry & Claire Steinberg
Hope and Roy Turney
Kent Valandra
Dorothy Wagle
Diane & Ernie Wolfe III
and Private Collectors

PREFACE

The California Heritage Museum and "Masks of the World"

Built in 1894 by the nationally renown architect Sumner P. Hunt for Roy Jones, the son of Santa Monica's founder, Senator John P. Jones, the California Heritage Museum has been open to the public since 1980. Rather than commemorate only the life of the Jones family, the Heritage Museum is committed to preserve the entire area's history. Thus the Historic Landmark building became a California history museum, not just a historic house. Community programming includes unique and innovative rotating exhibitions, lectures, workshops, and concerts.

The Museum's Mission is to present displays of American decorative and fine arts and to promote the passion that is collecting. Depression glass, California pottery, quilts, Hawaiana, surfboards, Mexican pottery, Arts and Crafts Movement furniture and pottery, Plein Aire landscape paintings, eventually become a unique exhibition at the Museum, usually in room settings that encourage the visitor to begin (if they have not already started), their own exciting collection.

Under the guidance of guest curator Jim Pieper, thirty collectors lent more than 350 masks to the second floor *"Masks of the World"* exhibition. The masks were organized by country and continent and represented a wide variety of masking traditions. Many of the local Los Angeles and Santa Monica schools made excellent use of this exhibition by bringing students to draw the masks, and in many instances, to make their own masks as classroom projects.

Tobi Smith, Executive Director, May, 1999

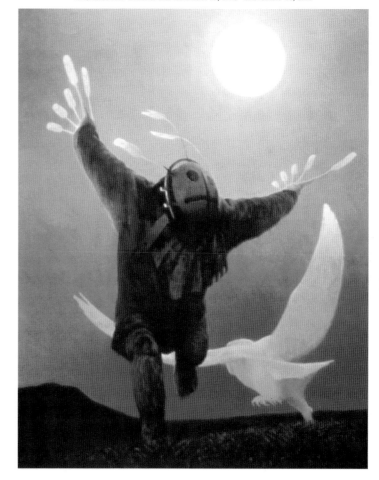

THE CALIFORNIA HERITAGE MUSEUM PRESENTS

MASKS OF THE WORLD

EXHIBITION DATES: SEPTEMBER 19, 1998 - JANUARY 10, 1999

INTRODUCTION Jim Pieper

How Did Masking Start?

Humankind's first crafted mask appeared thousands of years ago arising from the need for camouflage for the hunt. Animal hide was used to cover and blend the hunter with the environment.

As the hunter and his society evolved, their perception of their surroundings was tinged with an awareness of the spiritual, the mysteries of life. Faced with this newfound sensitivity, humans slowly began to seek the aid of simple amulets and rituals to help them cope with the world. Animal parts, claw, teeth, skulls and hide were among these early ritual objects. Hide draped over the face aided the participant to blend the animal spirit with his own mind and body, taking on the persona, power and spirit of the animal.

As time passed, fertility, harvest, healing, war, satire, theater...the life forces of society were encapsulated into the presence of these coverings of the face. In transforming the physical appearance, the mask allowed the wearer the potential of modifying his very essence and spirit. In the act of changing his outward image, he became spirit filled and feel the empowerment of a god, or, in contrast, infused with bizarre behavior as an uncontrolled clown. The mask wearer was not limited. He needed no longer to be himself. The mask gave him the permission to be anything and act in any way he chose.

This primary use of the mask, which still touches nearly every corner of the earth, has evolved, being influenced by the religious mythologies and ethos of society. Some masking traditions, however, remain pure to their ancient origins. In the dances of the Pueblo Indians of the United States a total blending of the masked individual with the ancient spirit they represent is experienced. In New Guinea masks decorate yams (the vegetable) and call on ancestral spirits to benefit village fertility.

We only have to look at Bali and Java to see the influence of Hindu deities. Tibet shows us the protectors and the divinity of Buddhism. The design forms of Africa are frequently interpreted to have extensive Muslim influences.

Christianity arrived in the new world with Alvarado and Coronado in the 1500's. They introduced the Dance of the Conquest and the Dance of the Moors and Christians, both telling the old story of good's triumph over evil, interpreted as Christianity triumphing over the pagans. In Chiapas, Mexico, the prehistoric Dance of the Deer had two figures added by the invading Christians and it became the Dance of David and Goliath. Overlay after overlay, new mythologies continue, influencing and changing the earlier primary ritual.

Masking is a cloaking device for society where even kings could become commoners for a night. The figure of the doctor (dottore) joined the Carnival of Venice from the pages of history, as one who examined the bodies of the plague victims in Europe. Today the evolution continues as we see Mickey Mouse enter the world of ceremony and ritual in Africa and the Americas. The future is only limited by the mind's creativity, and maybe the world of spirits it touches.

You are about to view over 350 masks representing many cultures of the world, but this is only a representative scratch on the surface of the totality of the world's masking ritual.

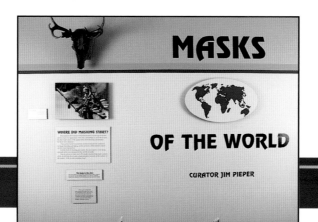

The EXHIBIT

MASKS OF THE WORLD

CURATOR JIM PIEPER

The Entry

The visitors to the Masks of the World exhibit were greeted by an ancient deer mask. Natural objects were likely among the first masks used by human beings in an attempt to harness the skills and spirits of the animals. To this day many of these basic motives remain unchanged. Whether it is the simple child's mask at halloween or the intricate mask of an African tribal ritual, the mask represents a transformation. It allows the wearer to be someone or something they are not.

So it is that the warrior in the painting at the beginning of the show wears the wolf mask as he prepares for battle. In the wearing the warrior calls forth the cunning and courage of the great predator to be with him and in him in the conflict that follows.

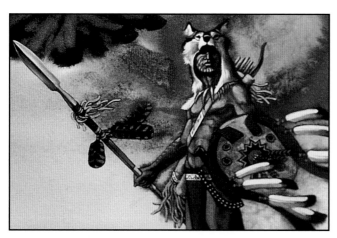

Deer Dance Mask
The deer is ceremonially killed, then worn in a dance that blends Christianity with ancient ways. This ceremony is performed on Saint Peter and Saint John days. The deer's killing is ritually reenacted. The deer is then touched to obtain the power of the Mountain Spirit. Deer skull, fur, antler, 12 inches.
Cotopoxi, Ecuador
Ca. late 20th century
Collection of Jim and Jeanne Pieper

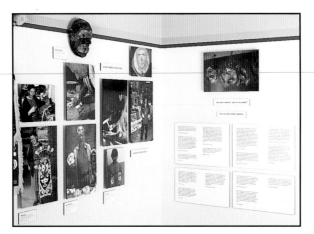

The California Heritage Museum has always celebrated collectors and their collections. Their shows have drawn upon these treasures, always dependent upon the generosity of the lenders. So it is that the Masks of the World exhibit was derived from the masks of many collectors, people who have experienced the beauty and power of the masking tradition, and have filled their homes with these beautiful objects. Many of them shared their thoughts about masks and why they were attracted to collecting them. As the visitor turned the corner at the entry these thoughts were shared with them. You will find their comments sprinkled throughout this book.

Mask Making: Materials and Methods

Masks can be made from almost anything, from the animal fur or skulls to discarded tin cans. The materials and methods the skilled mask makers used to create their "magic" were explored as the visitor moved deeper into the exhibit. Visitors encountered both the makers and their products, and captured a sense of the creative processes at work around the world.

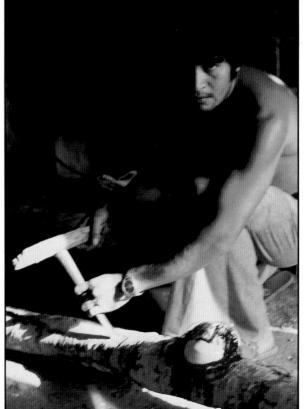

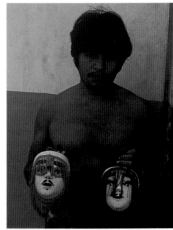

Sr. Gutierrez proudly holding two of his carnival masks. These mask are sold in Ocozocoaotla in direct competition with molded clay masks.
Photo: Jim Pieper

Mexicano Masks
Dance of the Mexicanos masks hang from the roof of a *Moreria*, the organization that rents masks for celebrations.
Guatemala
1980s
Photo: Jim Pieper

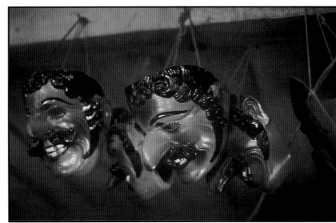

Antonio Gutierrez carves wooden masks on the dirt floor of his small house.
Ocozocoaotla, Chiapas, Mexico
1983
Photo: Jim Pieper

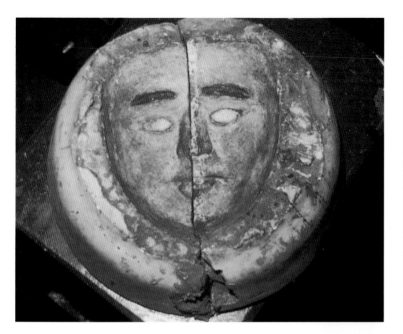

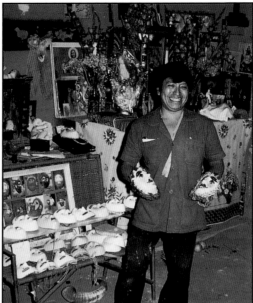

Molded Clay Masks
This mask maker competes against Antonio Gutierrez, who makes small wood masks in the same town. These masks are formed in a two-part clay mold. They represent one of the few applications of clay or ceramic masks used in Mexican ceremonies.
Ocozocoaotla, Chiapas, Mexico
1980s
Photo: Jim Pieper

Papier-mâché Masks
Masks are formed over crude mud molds. This is Anzelmo Circiro making molds.
Ayutla, Guerrero, Mexico
1980s
Photo: Jim Pieper

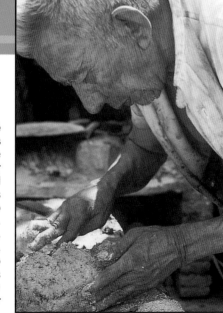

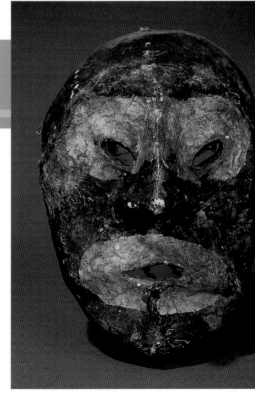

Soldier or Judas Mask
Papier-mâché mask that would have been used during Lenten ceremonies. They are normally destroyed at the conclusion of the ceremony. 9 inches.
Cora People
Nayarit, Mexico
Ca. late 20th century
Collection of Larry and Sandy Roseman

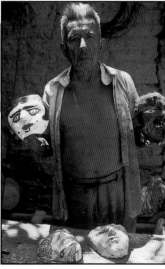

Sr. Circiro holding two of his masks.
Ayutla, Guerrero, Mexico
1980s
Photo: Jim Pieper

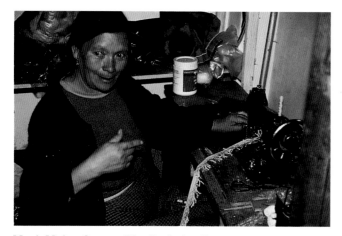

Mask Maker Senora Rita Profetisa Ermosa at work.
Ecuador
1995
Photo: Jim Pieper

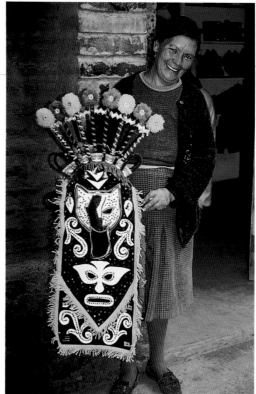

Senora Ermosa holding one
of her *Diablo Umo* masks.
Ecuador
1995
Photo: Jim Pieper

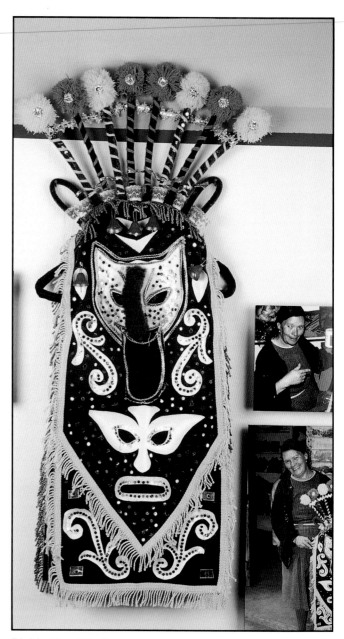

Diablo Umo Mask
Made by Senora Ermosa.
Ecuador
1995
Collection of Jim and Jeanne Pieper

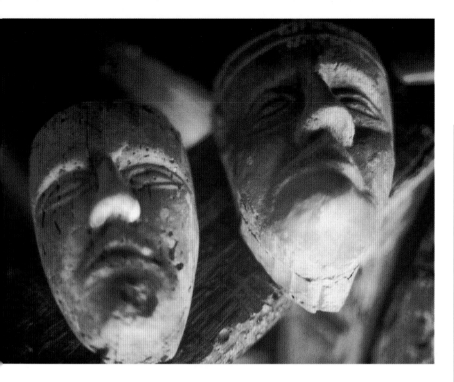

Above:
Wire Mask Molds
Wooden molds are used to form screen masks of the Chinelo.
Morelos, Mexico 1980s
Photo: Jim Pieper

Right:
Sr. Villamiel forms screen over a wooden mold. He then shapes the screen, paints it and attaches a woven horsehair beard and hair to complete the mask of Chinelo.
Photo: Jim Pieper

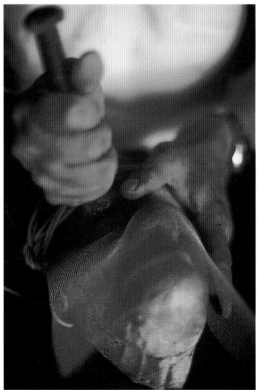

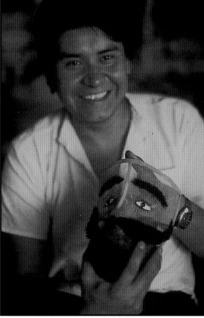

Rubin Villamiel is a fourth generation mask maker.
Photo: Jim Pieper

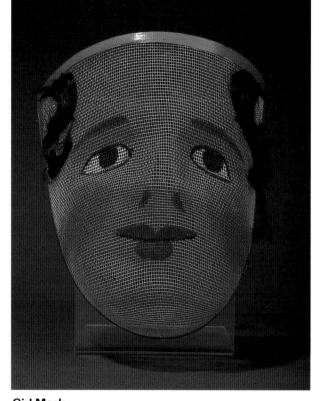

Girl Mask
Painted wire mesh, and human hair, 6.5 inches.
Salcedo, Cotopaxi, Ecuador
Ca. late 20th century
Collection of Hope and Roy Turney

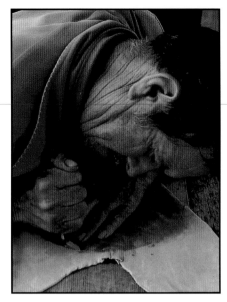

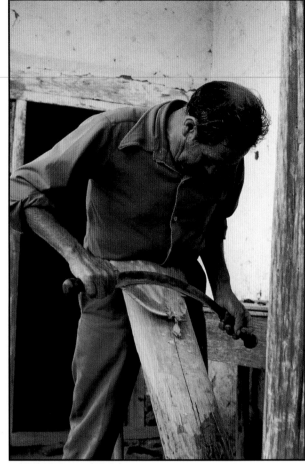

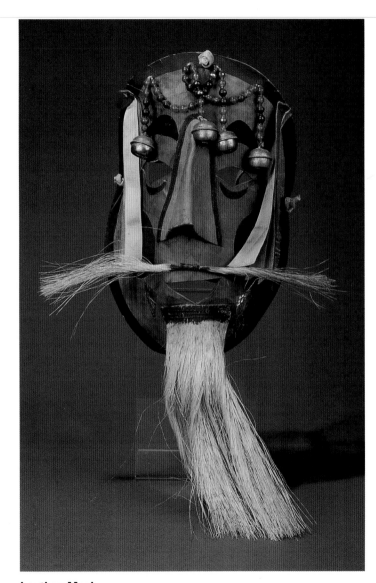

Leather Mask Making

Juan Jose Aquilar is a third generation mask maker shown forming a cowhide mask. The work takes about one-and-a-half days to complete. He begins by cutting the mask shape and thinning the hide. Then he adds the features. About half the masks he creates are sold through a local tourist shop. The other half are sold for the ceremonies.
Tzotzil People
Huixtan, Chiapas, Mexico
1987
Photo: Jim Pieper

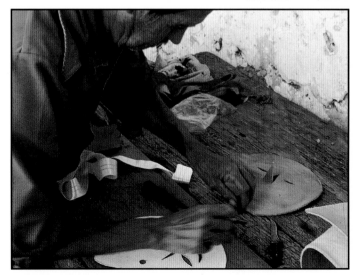

Leather Mask

Mask maker, Gregorio Ballinas.
Huistan, Chiapas, Mexico
Ca. 1974
Collection of Ann and Monroe Morgan

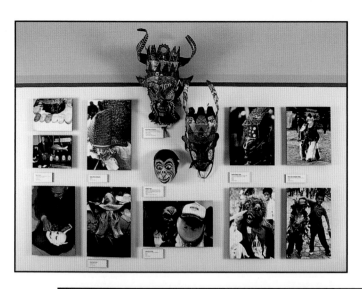

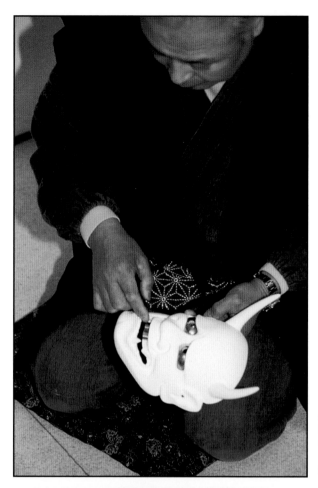

Japanese mask maker at work.
Kyoto, Japan.
1990s
Photo: Jim Pieper

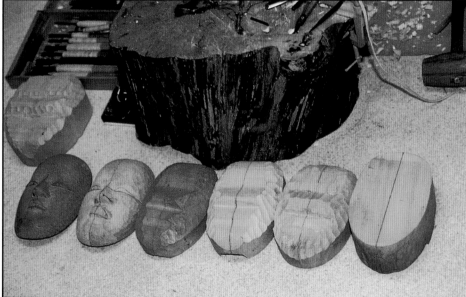

The progress of the wooden mask
through various stages of carving.
Kyoto, Japan
1990s
Photo: Jim Pieper

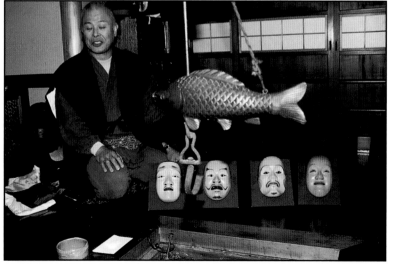

Mask maker with
some of his creations.
Kyoto, Japan
1990s
Photo: Jim Pieper

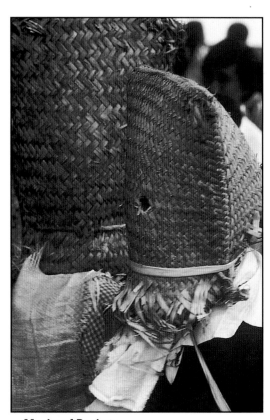

Masks of Baskets
Mexico
1990s
Photo: Jim Pieper

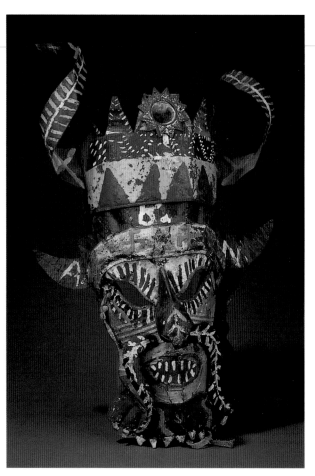

Tin Masks
These two masks are made of tin cans and are danced in *12 Pares De Francia* (Lords of France). The dance reflects the royalty of France. Tin and wire, 21 inches and 22 inches.
Queretaro, Mexico
Ca. mid-20th century
Collection of Jim and Jeanne Pieper

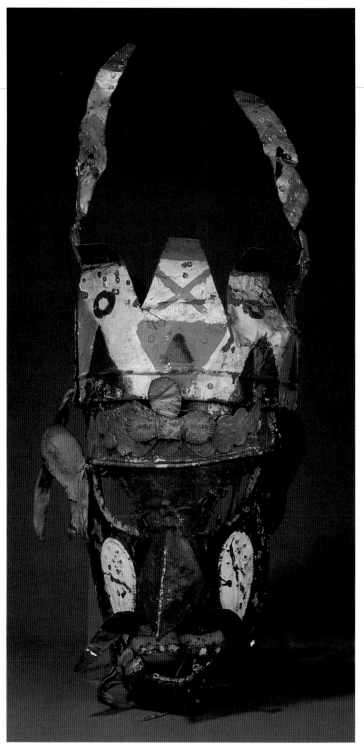

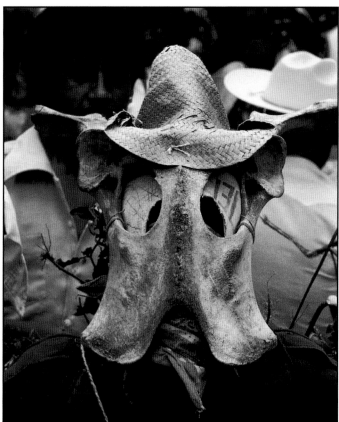

Bone Mask
Chichiculatco, Guerrero,
Mexico
1980s
Photo: Jim Pieper

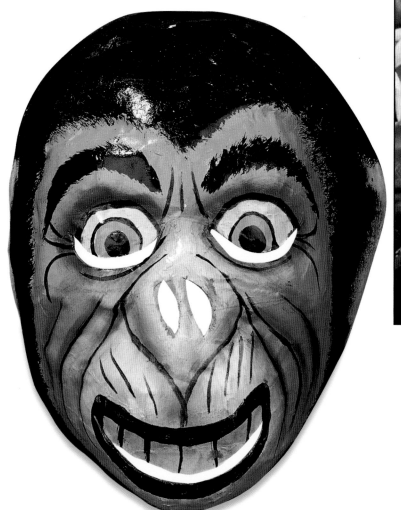

Monkey Mask
Molded paper, 8 inches.
Cayambe, Ecuador
Ca. 1995
*Collection of Jim and
Jeanne Pieper*

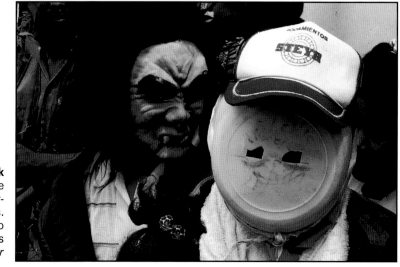

Tupperware Mask
A little creative
thinking can gener-
ate wonders.
Mexico
1990s
Photo: Jim Pieper

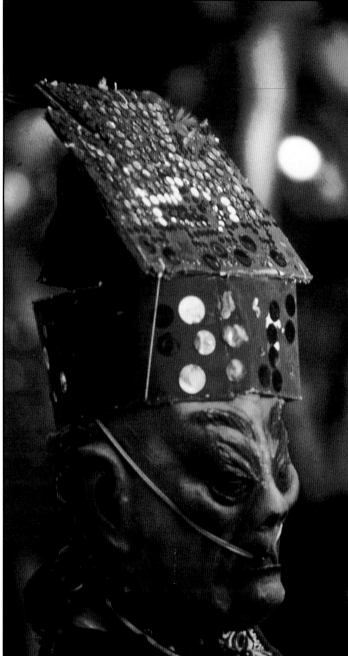

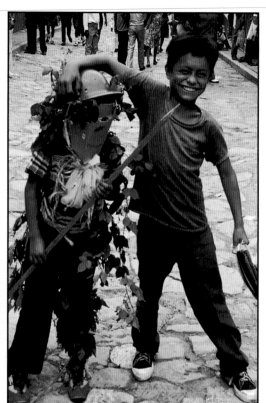

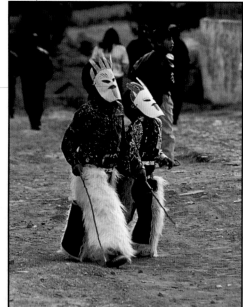

Above & left:
Paper and Corrugated Masks
These home made masks allow everyone
to be creative and join the festivities.
Mexico
1990s
Photo: Jim Pieper

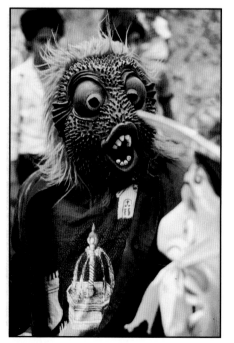

Contemporary Mask
Corrugated cardboard and rubber.
Puebla, Mexico
Ca. 1980s
Photo: Jim Pieper

Molded Rubber Mask
This is a very popular
material for masks
today. The masks are
molded in both the
United States and
Mexico.
Mexico
1990s
Photo: Jim Pieper

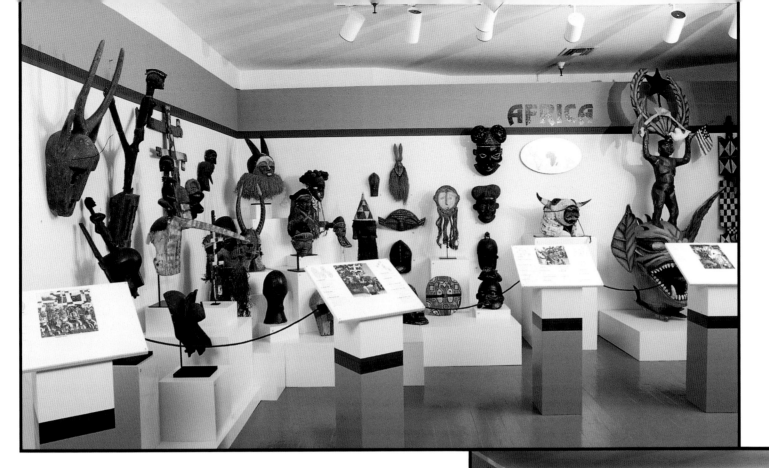
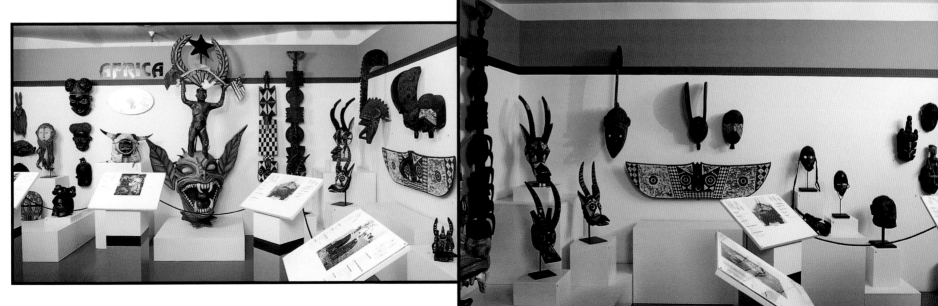

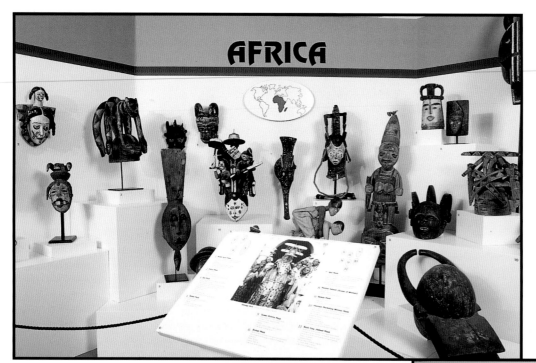

AFRICA

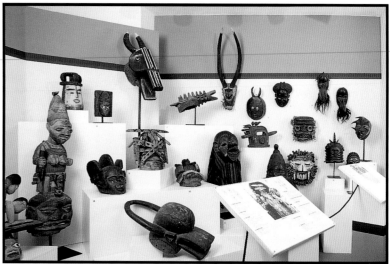

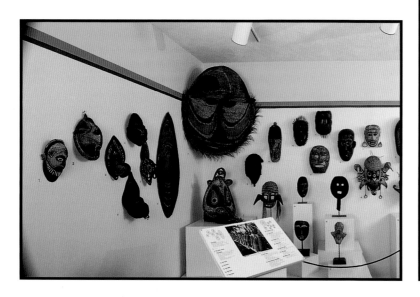

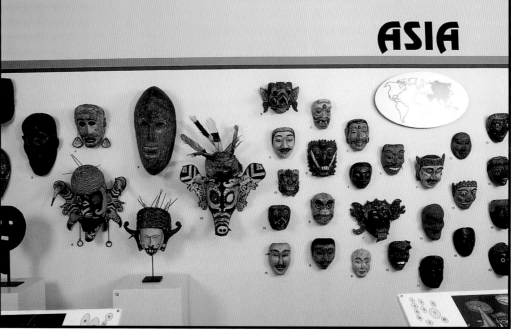

ASIA

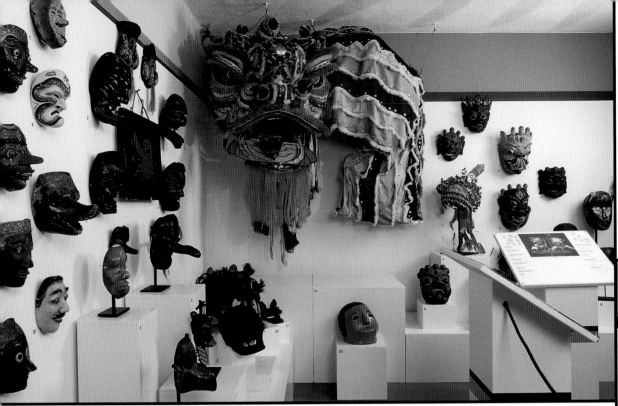

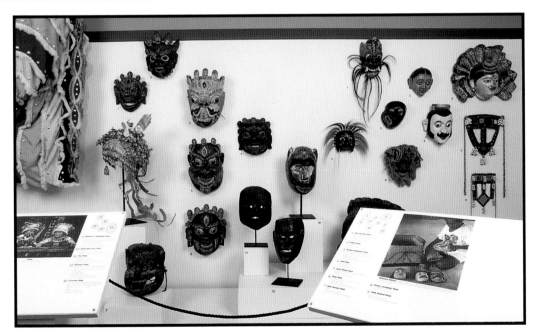

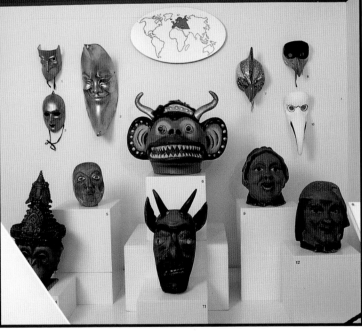

EUROPE

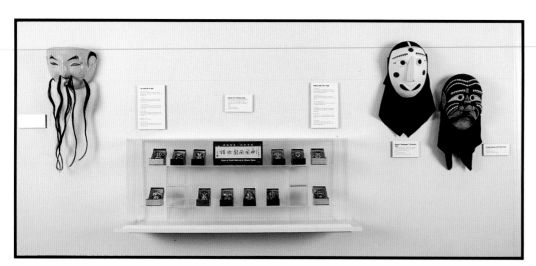

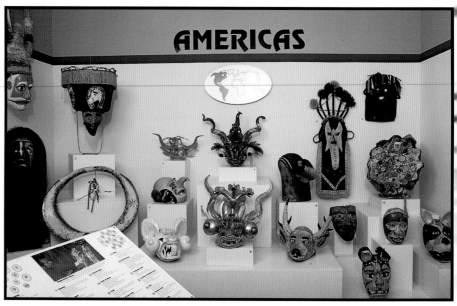

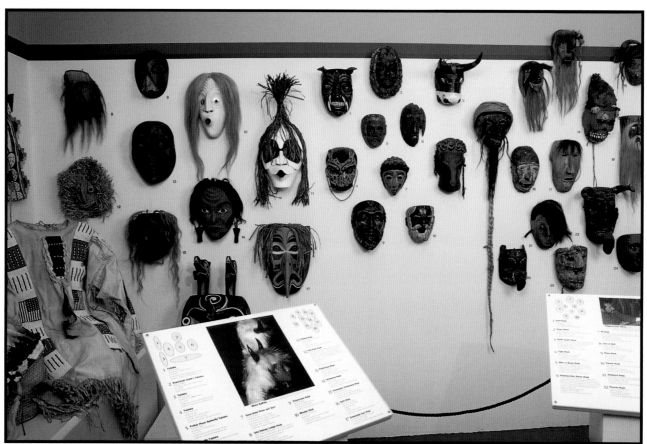

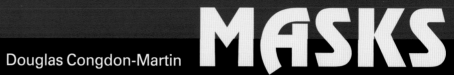

MASKS

Douglas Congdon-Martin

Several months after the Masks of the World exhibit had closed, one of the fine docents of the California Heritage Museum confessed to me that she had had some misgivings about the show. In the morning, when she was alone in the museum unlocking doors and turning on lights in preparation for the exhibit's visitors, she had felt uneasy in the company of the masks.

It was an understandable reaction. The masks have a powerful presence. Since prehistoric times they have been an integral part of human rituals. Masked dancers are found painted on walls of caves from over 25000 years ago. Masks adorned the dead in Egypt's pyramids and in burial sites of ancient Peruvians. They are found in all times, including our own, on every continent, and in nearly every culture. Wherever they appear they are invested with a certain power. Their uses range from profoundly spiritual to delightfully playful, from masked demons to masked heroes.

The power of the masks comes not from their outward beauty, though they are often extraordinarily crafted, but from the layers of tradition, myth, and belief that lie behind them. Masks carry the ancient stories of tribe and nation. They are embodiments of ancestors and gods. They are used in dances that reenact the significant moments of the race, moments that range from the foundation of the universe, to hard won battle victories, to success in the hunt or the harvest.

In all of this, masks help define the group or tribe, and the individual's place within it. They are used to ritualize the passing of the seasons. Around the world you will find them used to mark the planting and harvesting, the beginning of spring and the coming of winter. They play a part in religious ceremonies, and, as we see at Mardi Gras and Halloween, the masks continue to be used even when their original spiritual impetus is lost in the mists of time. And at those most profoundly personal moments–births, circumcisions, passages into adolescence and adulthood, marriages, and funerals–masks represent the presence of the holy and of ancestors.

It is remarkable how similarly masks are used in divergent cultures, separated by time and place. That commonality of practice and some uncanny likenesses of form tempt one to look for ethnographic links to make sense of it all. Experts warn against it, finding no evidence of a direct relationship between the cultures. The human connectedness, however, is another matter. What binds us and gives rise to certain commonality between the masks of the world is our need to make sense of the mysteries of the world, to concretize them, and, in doing so, to gain some measure of control over them.

Masks permit this. In donning the mask, the wearer partakes of the reality it represents. He becomes, to some degree, the ancestor, god, or animal carved into the mask, and often he acts out the life of that being in a dance or ritual drama. It is not unlike a great actor, who, under a mask of grease paint and wig, for a brief hour or two takes on the *persona* of the character he or she is portraying. If the actors are skilled, we suspend disbelief and allow ourselves to accept them for the ones they purport to be, letting them move us to tears and laughter. By this we are permitting ourselves to be transformed by their performance, much as the tribal people are transformed by the dances and ritual drama that accompany these masks.

That word, *persona*, is interesting. It is the Latin word for mask, and the source of the English word "personality," which, like the mask, is that aspect of ourselves that we show to others. Etymologically, then, we all wear masks. As healthy human beings our masks tend to be pretty much the same in every segment of our lives, with some variations for our roles as worker, spouse, parent, or child. At certain times or in certain conditions other sides of our personalities, other masks, emerge to help us cope with new or threatening challenges in our environment. This is a key element in our adaptability, which, as long as we can maintain a unified self behind the masks, can aid us in our struggle for survival.

Perhaps, then, at its root the universality of masks is personal as much as cultural. Masks grow out of the common human striving for meaning, for belonging, for survival. They exist because of the uniquely human ability to feel empathy, to take on the feelings, perceptions, even the personality of another being, be it god, spirit, ancestor, or animal, and in doing so move us to a deeper level of understanding and empowerment.

Nearly all of the masks in the Masks of the World exhibit and in this book have been "danced," which is a way of saying they have had an authentic part in the lives of the people who created them. This is of importance to collectors, of course, because so many masks are being carved today expressly for sale to those who admire their artistry. But it also adds to the sense of power these objects embody. They have been used. They have absorbed the sweat and tears of their wearers. The religious masks have been lovingly covered with the soil of the earth or the blood of sacrifice. They have carried the spirits of ancestors, told the stories of the people, made real the presence of the holy. The festive masks have brought joy to the lives of the revellers and retold the stories that forged them into a people. The theatrical masks have turned mere mortals into immortal characters, bringing to life the timeless stories of the human experience.

Because of the important place masks have in the culture, the artistry employed in their creation is often quite exquisite. Mask makers are often a revered member of the society, undergoing years of apprenticeship and education to refine their art. Their genius is attested to by the number of great 20th century

Western painters and sculptors who were influenced by the masks of Africa and elsewhere. These masks, even devoid of their functionality, continue to touch our aesthetic sensibilities. And when they are viewed in the total context of their creation, we find them even more wonderful and powerful to behold.

Organization and Tribal Names

The book, like the exhibit, is organized by regions. Within each region, the masks are organized by country. In fact, masks are more commonly associated with tribes than nations, and tribes often cross national boundaries. The spelling of tribal names presents a challenge to the researcher, especially when the objects and information about them come from a variety of sources. We strove for consistency, choosing what seemed the most commonly accepted spelling, and referring to the *Encyclopedia of World Cultures*, Timothy J. O'Leary and David Levinson, editors (Boston, G.K. Hall & Co., 1991) when necessary.

Reference Abbreviations Used in Descriptions

These reference abbreviations are used in descriptions, followed by page numbers (p.) or plate numbers (pl.). Please refer to the Bibliography for a complete description of the works cited.

Bruggmann: Bruggmann & Gerber. *Indians of the Northwest Coast*
Bushell NM: Bushell. *Netsuke Masks*
Colton: Colton. *Hopi Kachina Dolls*
Goonatilleka MMSSL: Goonatilleka. *Masks and Mask Systems of Sri Lanka*
Jacobsen CF: Jacobson & Fritz. *Changing Faces*
Jonaitis: Jonaitis. *From the Land of the Totem Poles*
Mack MAME: Mack. *Masks and the Art of Expression*
Madsic PANG: Maksic & Meskil. *Primitive Art of New Guinea*
Segy ASS: Segy. *African Sculpture Speaks*
Segy MBA: Segy. *Masks of Black Africa*
Sieber AACL: Sieber & Walker. *African Art in the Cycle of Life*
Song MSUT: Song. *Minsok sajin ukpyolchan torots (Korean Masks)*
TSW: Seattle Art Museum. *The Spirit Within*
Willett AA: Willett. *African Art*
Wright: Wright. *Hopi Kachinas*

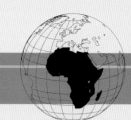

AFRICA

GUINEA BISSAU

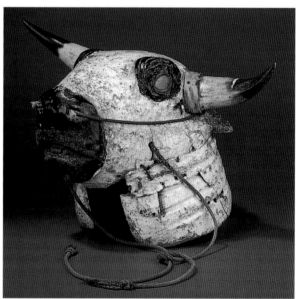

Bull Helmet Mask
Cabarao Society initiation mask. Danced by the oldest members of this secret society representing their final matriculation from earlier fish form head dresses to the terrestrially based cows and bulls. Wood, bottle glass eyes, horn, fabric, leather, and rope, 16 inches.
Bidjogo Islands, Guinea Bissau
Collection of Ed Moses

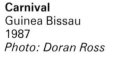

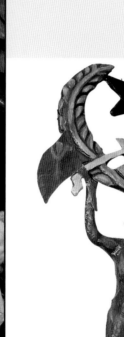

Carnival
Guinea Bissau
1987
Photo: Doran Ross

Carnival Mask
Often the masks from this one-time Portuguese colony are thematic or political. This example, from February, 1989, celebrates the belief that the Bissauan leadership, through their offices, could bring *détente* to the United States and Russia. Later the same year the Berlin wall came down and the Cold War ended. Papier-mâché, 90 inches.
Guinea Bissau
Ca. 1980s
Collection of Diane and Ernie Wolfe III

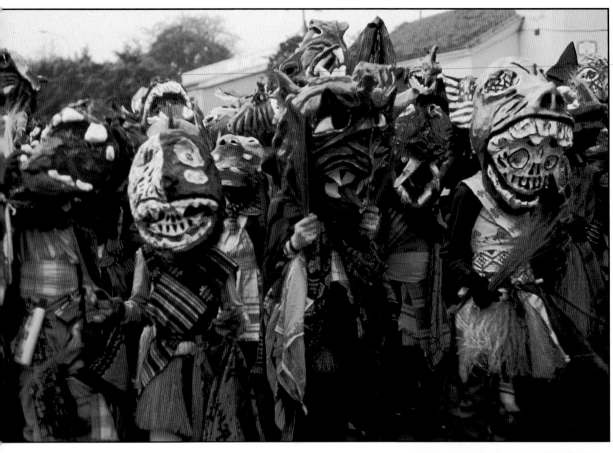

Carnival
Guinea Bissau
1987
Photos: Doran Ross

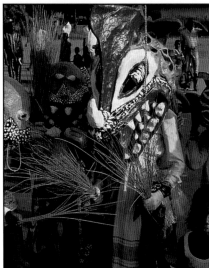

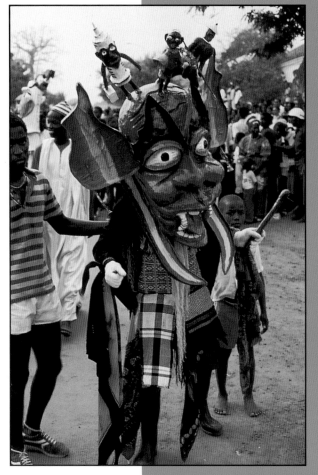

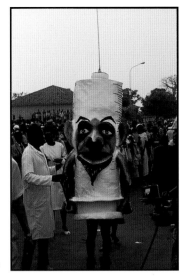

Carnival
Guinea Bissau
1987
Photos: Doran Ross

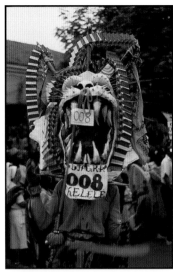

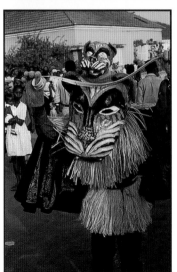

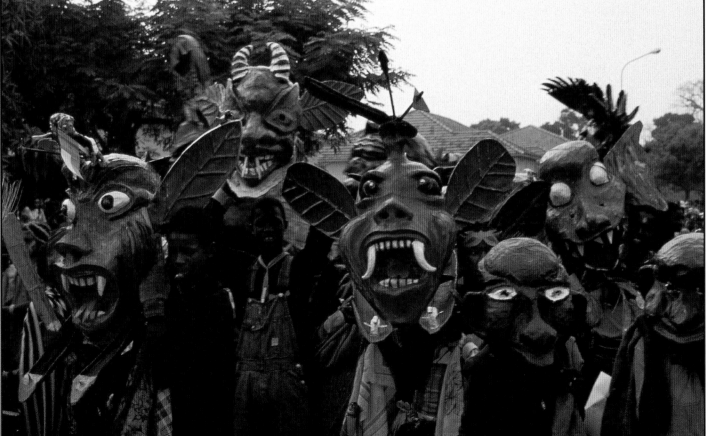

25

MALI

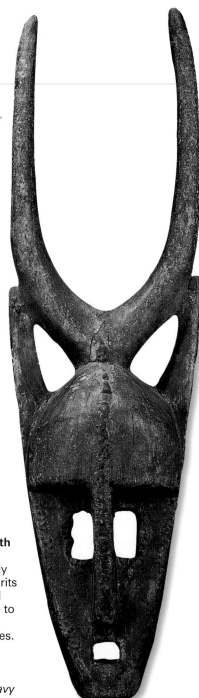

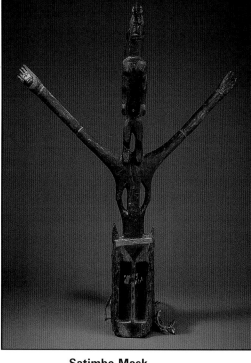

Satimbe Mask
Antelope surmounted by human form. The figure represents Yasigine, the only woman admitted to the Awa male society *(Segy, MBA, pl. 16).* Polychrome wood, fiber, and cowry shell, 39 inches.
Dogon People
Mali
Collection of Dr. Harry and Claire Steinberg

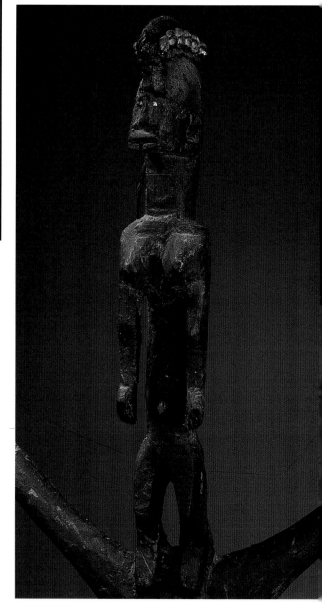

Kore Society Mask with Horns
This mask is particularly concerned with the spirits who attack the sky and thus bring rain to earth to provide fertility to the fields. Wood, 32.5 inches.
Bambara people
Mali
Ca. 19th century
Collection of Woods Davy

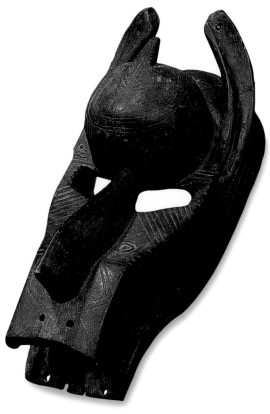

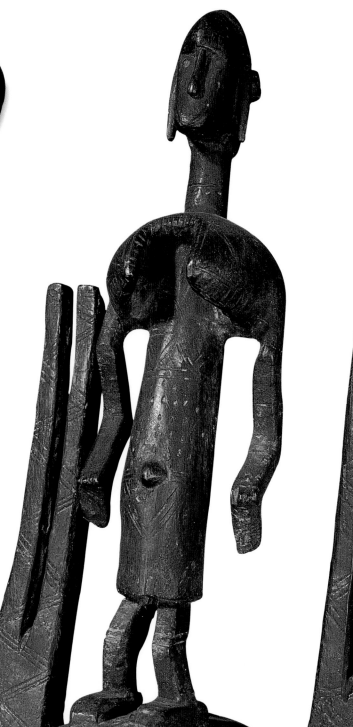

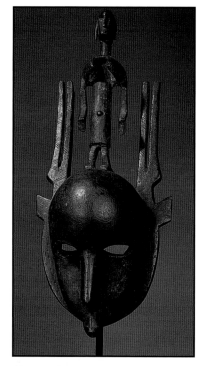

Bambara Kore Hyena Mask
The hyena is the protective guardian of the Kore Society, a group principally involved in agricultural activities, such as ceremonies at planting and for rain *(Segy, ASS, p. 150-151)*. Wood, 14.75 inches.
Bambara Kore Society
Mali
Ca. 20th century
Collection of Jerry Solomon, Los Angeles

N'tomo Mask
At the center of this mask is a female ancestor figure. The mask was used in ceremonies of the N'tomo Society for men. The Bambara men are organized by age groups with members progressing from one group to the next as they mature. *(Segy, ASS, p. 150).* N'tomo (or Ndomo) is for the uncircumcised pre-teens, who spend five years in this stage, going through five levels of instruction. At the end they are circumcised *(Sieber, AACL, p. 52).* Wood, 21.75 inches.
Bambara N'tomo Society
Mali
Ca. 20th century
Collection of Jerry Solomon, Los Angeles

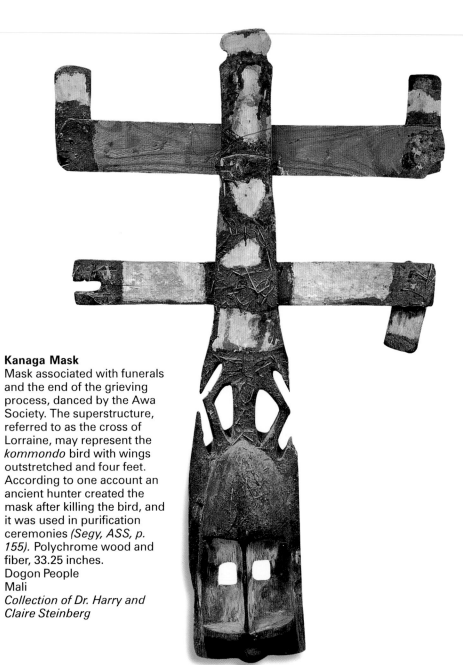

Kanaga Mask
Mask associated with funerals and the end of the grieving process, danced by the Awa Society. The superstructure, referred to as the cross of Lorraine, may represent the *kommondo* bird with wings outstretched and four feet. According to one account an ancient hunter created the mask after killing the bird, and it was used in purification ceremonies *(Segy, ASS, p. 155)*. Polychrome wood and fiber, 33.25 inches.
Dogon People
Mali
Collection of Dr. Harry and Claire Steinberg

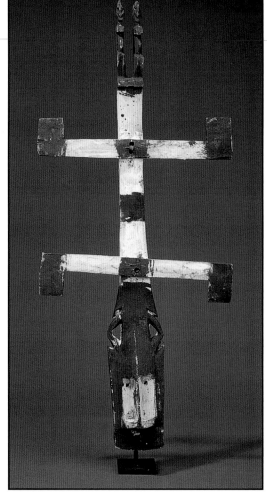

Kanaga Mask
The figures at the top of this mask represent the original Dogon couple. Polychrome wood, and wire, 22.5 inches.
Dogon People
Mali
Ca. mid-20th century
Collection of Joni and Monte Gordon, Newspace, Los Angeles

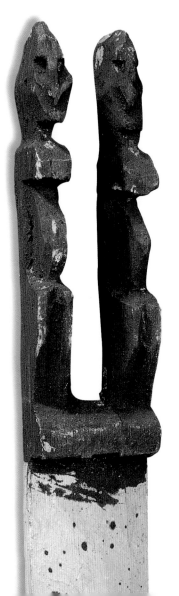

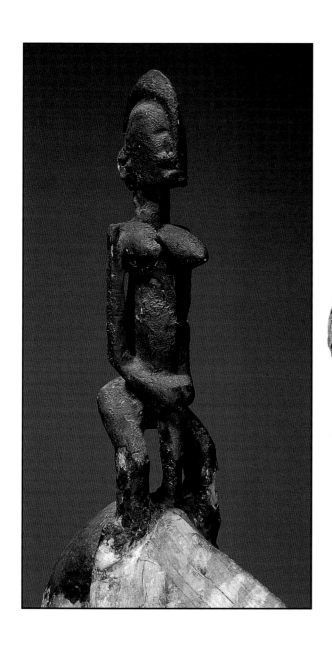

We pursue and collect African art for the joy, beauty and mystery we find in the objects, and for their standards of abstracted form that have greatly influenced twentieth century Western art.
Dr. Richard and Jan Baum

Hornbill Mask
Surmounted by female figure, danced during funeral ceremonies and special death anniversary ceremonies. Polychrome wood, 28.25 inches.
Dogon people
Bandiagara Cliffs, Central Mali
Ca. early to mid-20th century
Collection of Woods Davy

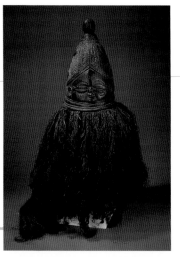

Sowei Helmet Mask

The Sande Women's society took in girls as they reached puberty and instructed them in the duties that would be required of them in adulthood. Segy reports that perspective husbands often paid the initiation fee to the society. The rings at the neck are, according to Segy, "fat rings" which symbolize the maturing into womanhood. After training, the woman received a new name. *(Segy, ASS, pp. 161-163).* Wood and natural fiber, 14.5 inches (head only). Mende People
Sierra Leone/Liberia
Collection of Dr. Harry and Claire Steinberg

SIERRA LEONE

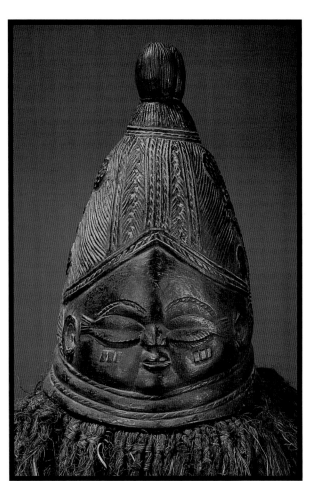

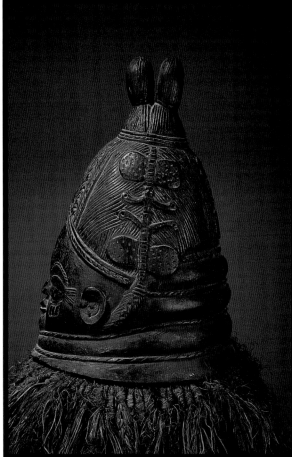

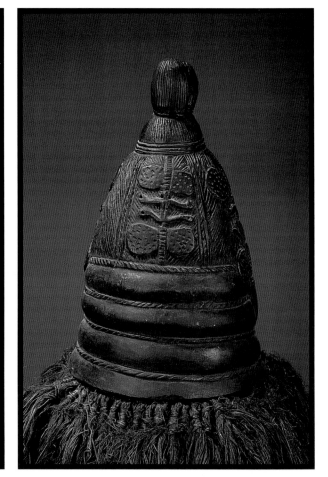

LIBERIA

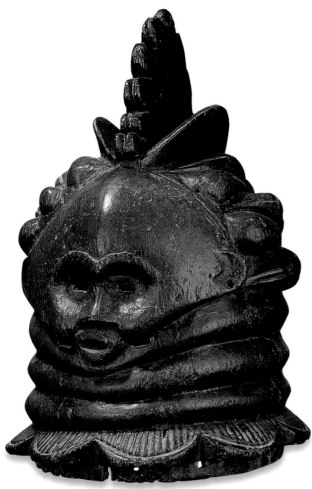

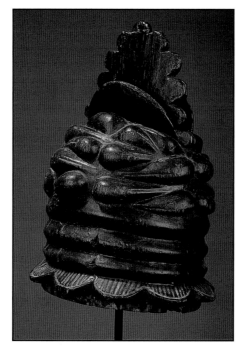

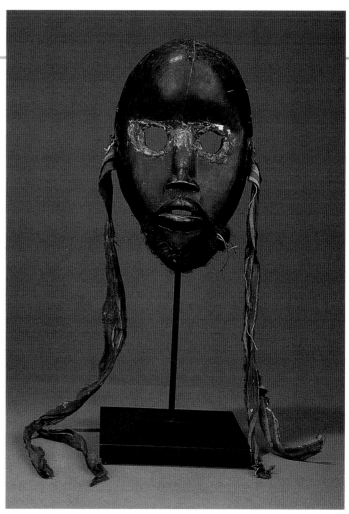

Women's Sande Society Helmet Mask
Similar to that found in Sierra Leone, this too was a mask of the Women's Secret Sande Society, formed to instruct young girls into the ways of womanhood. Unusual in African cultures, these masks are worn by women, though carved by men. *(Sieber, AACL, p. 56)*. Wood, 13.5 inches.
Vai People
Southwestern Liberia
Ca. late 19th century
Collection of Woods Davy

Poro Society Mask
Masks served to enforce the tribal council's rules, exercising social control. Each mask may have a special interest, which can be seen more in the rest of the costume than in the mask itself *(Sieber, AACL, p.94)*. Polychrome wood, fiber, and fabric, 8.75 inches.
Dan People
Liberia
Ca. 20th century
Collection of Suzan Lerer

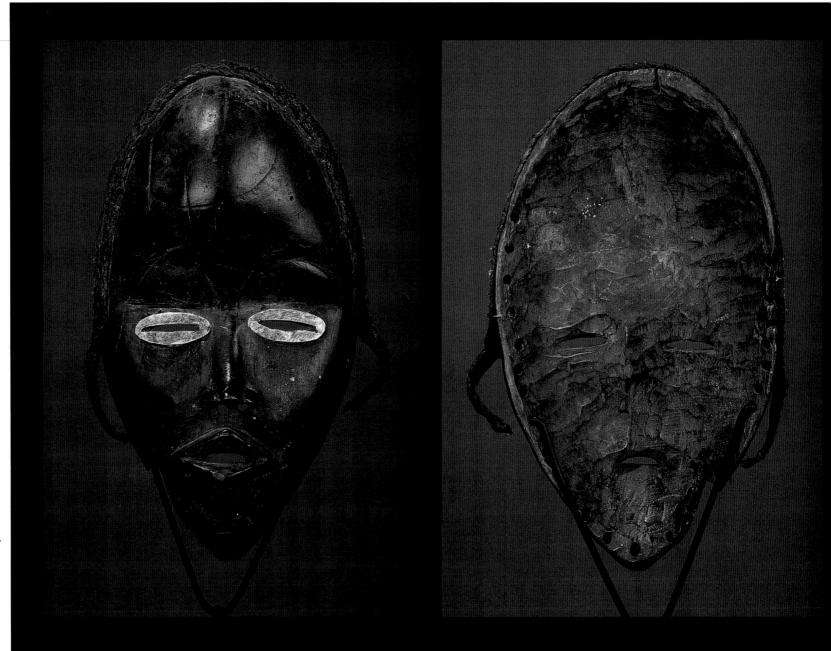

Dan Mask
Used for Poro Society
ritual : Wood, metal,
fiber, and hair, 8.5
inches.
Dan People
Ivory Coast or Liberia
Ca. 20th century
*Collection of Suzan
Lerer*

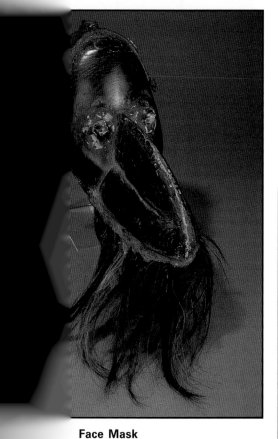

Face Mask
Used by those who collect
food for Guere festivals and
taxes to support the elders
(Segy, MBA, pl. 54-55).
Polychrome wood and
monkey hair, 13.5 inches.
Krahn People
Guere-Ouobe, Liberia
Ca. mid-20th century
*Collection of Helen Epstein,
Los Angeles*

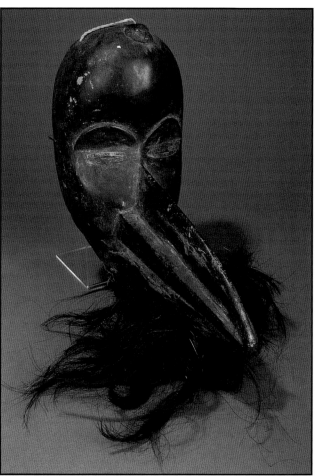

Face Mask
Polychrome wood, 9.5 inches.
Krahn People
Liberia.
Ca. early to mid 20th century
Collection of Joni and Monte Gordon, Newspace, Los Angeles

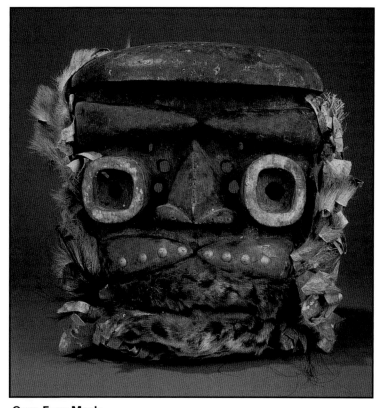

Ogre Face Mask
Wood, leather, fur, fiber, and tacks, 12 inches.
Guere People
Liberia
Collection of Dr. Harry and Claire Steinberg

Horned Mask

A Poro society mask. This mask
projects its power through the
multiple horns of the Duiker, a small
forest-dwelling antelope. The bells
under the nose suggest the mask's
use as a means to summon the power
of the forest. Wood, horn, mud, metal
bells, rope, and metal, 10.5 inches.
Guere People
Liberia
Ca. 2nd quarter 20th century
Collection of Diane and Ernie Wolfe III

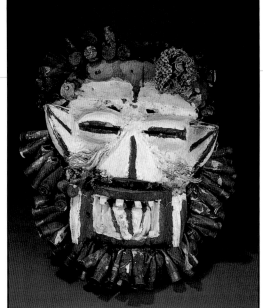

Face Mask

Chaser of evil spirits, empow-
ered by the shotgun shells
and protective medicine on its
forehead. Frequently used in
rites of passage, planting and
initiation. Wood, nails,
shotgun shells, bullets, hair
and hide, fabric, rope, and
fiber, 17.5 inches.
Guere People
Liberia
Ca. 2nd quarter 20th century
*Collection of Diane and Ernie
Wolfe III*

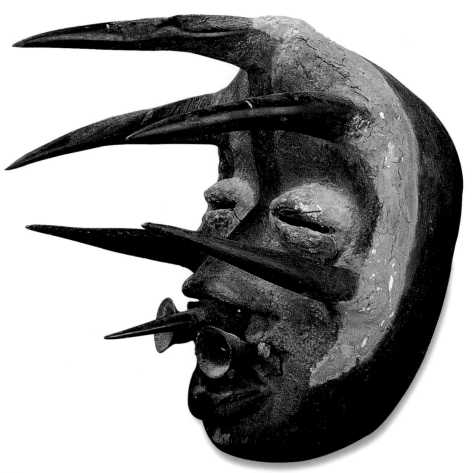

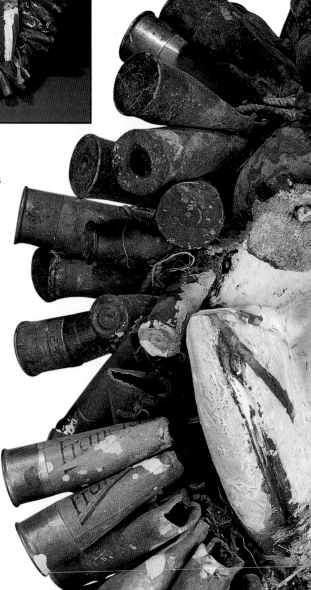

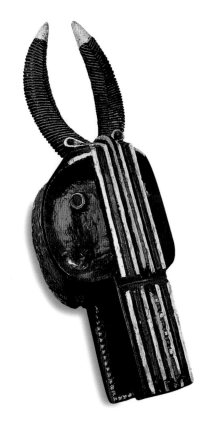

IVORY COAST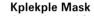

Goli Mask
Goli or *kakagye* masks represent the spirit of the dead *(Segy, ASS, pp. 64, 167-9)* and are associated with rites of passage such as birth and funerals. These masks are often repainted to redefine their power. Polychrome wood and fiber, 32 inches.
Baule People
Ivory Coast
Ca. early 20th century (ritually re-painted)
Collection of Diane and Ernie Wolfe III

Kplekple Mask
A mask used for commemoration, funerals, and community agricultural ceremonies at various seasons. *(Segy, ASS, p. 169).* Segy calls it "one of the great abstractions of African art" and explains that the roundness of the head represents the sun, and the horns the buffalo, "the symbol of fecundation." *(Segy, MBA, pl. 69).*
Polychrome wood, 16.5 inches.
Baule People
Ivory Coast
Collection of Dr. Harry and Claire Steinberg

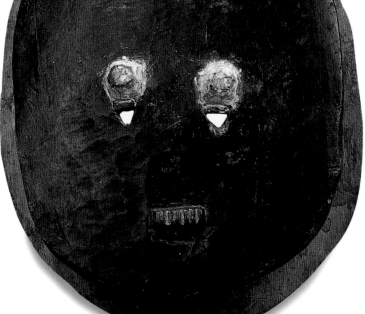

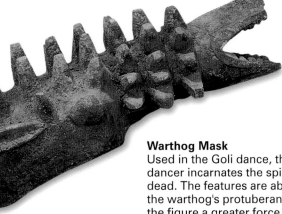

Warthog Mask
Used in the Goli dance, the masked dancer incarnates the spirit of the dead. The features are abstraction of the warthog's protuberances, giving the figure a greater force *(Segy, MBA, pl. 72).* Wood, 20.5 inches, front to back.
Baule People
Ivory Coast
Ca. early to mid 20th century
Collection of Woods Davy

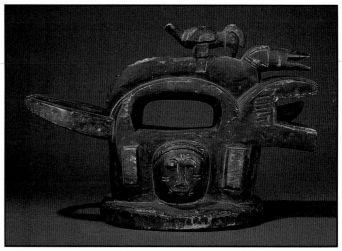

Antelope Mask
Polychrome wood, 11.75 inches.
Baule People
Ivory Coast
Collection of Dr. Harry and Claire Steinberg

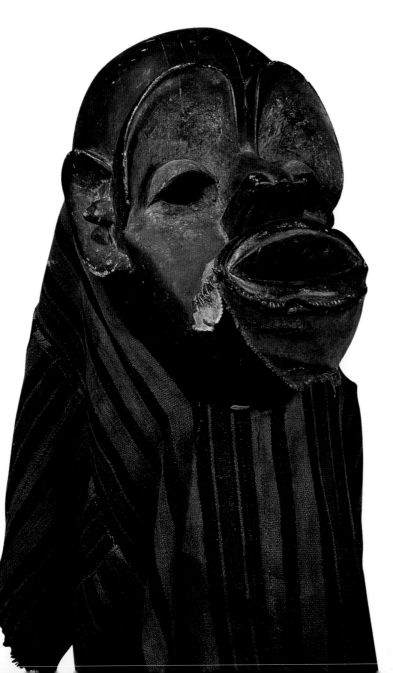

Monkey Mask
Wood, fabric, and skin, 15.5 inches (head only). Cultural use unknown Possibly Baule People
West Africa
Collection of Susan Lerer

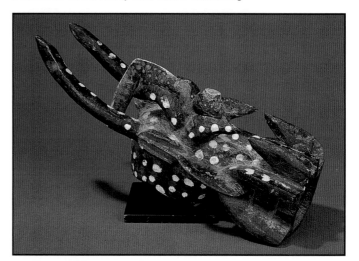

Waniougo Mask
With its crocodile jaws, antelope horns, and warthog tusks, this mask recalls the "chaotic conditions of the primordial world" *(Segy, ASS, p. 173).* Symbolizes power to recall mythical events in anti-witchcraft ceremonies. Polychrome wood, 13.75 inches.
Senufo People
Ivory Coast
Ca. mid 20th century
Collection of Helen Epstein, Los Angeles

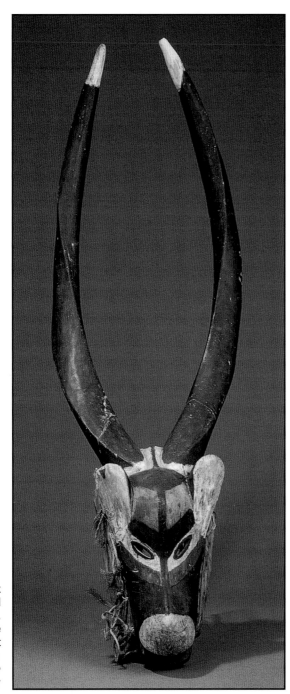

Antelope Mask
Polychrome wood
and fiber, 38 inches.
Guro People
Ivory Coast
*Collection of Dr.
Harry and Claire
Steinberg*

Female Face Mask
Wood, 12 inches.
Ivory Coast
*Collection of Dr. Harry
and Claire Steinberg*

The back of the mask shows the
exquisite skill of the carver.

BURKINA FASO

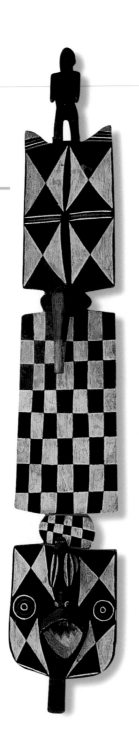

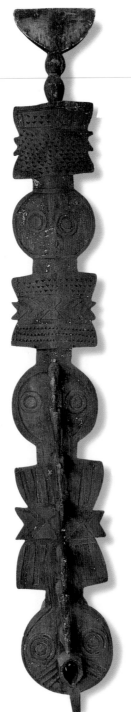

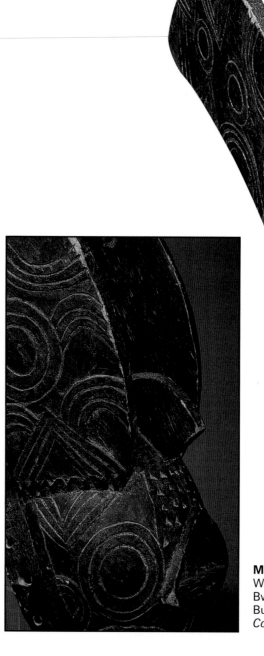

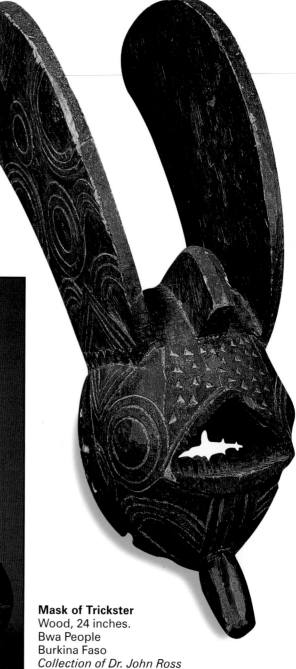

Right:
Plank Mask
Do Society mask, used in agricultural rituals *(Segy, ASS, p. 180)*. Polychrome wood, 59 inches.
Bwa People
Burkina Faso
Collection of Dr. Harry and Claire Steinberg

Far right:
Plank Mask
Harvest ceremonial mask.
Wood, 74 inches.
Bwa People
Burkina Faso
Ca. mid 20th century
Collection of Helen Epstein, Los Angeles

Mask of Trickster
Wood, 24 inches.
Bwa People
Burkina Faso
Collection of Dr. John Ross

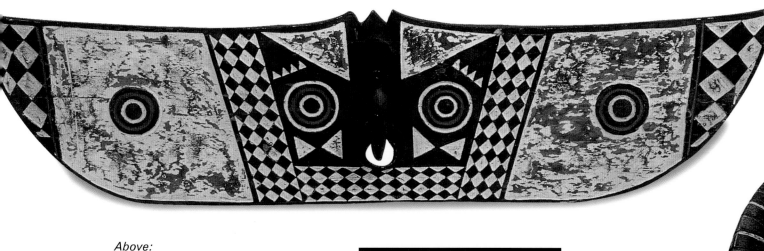

Above:
Hawk Mask
Others have called this "the bird of the night mask" *(Segy, MBA, pl. 115)* or the butterfly mask *(Willett, AA, p. 15)*. Polychrome wood, 51.25 inches wide.
Bwa People
Burkina Faso
Ca. mid 20th century
Collection of Helen Epstein, Los Angeles

Right:
Antelope Mask
Polychrome wood, 30 inches.
Bobo People
Koudougou region, Burkina Faso
Ca. 20th century
Collection of Suzan Lerer

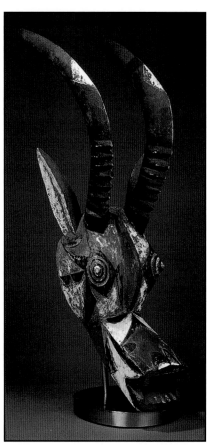

Female Koba Antelope Mask
Protective bush spirit associated with ancestor spirits. Wood and paint, 23.5 inches.
Nuna People
Tigan village, Upper Volta River Basin, Burkina Faso
Ca. mid 20th century
Collection of Woods Davy

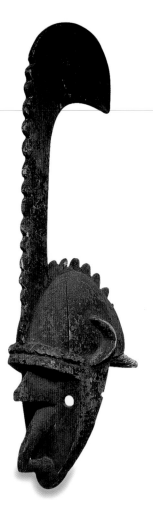

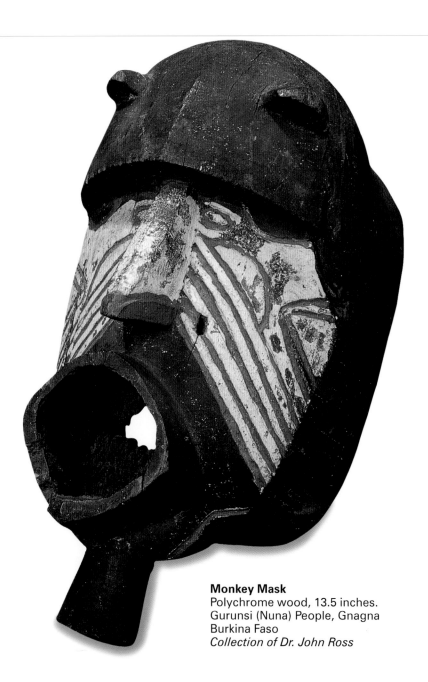

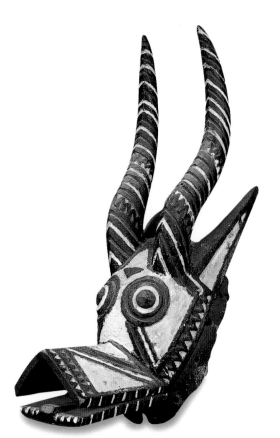

Zoomorphic Helmet Mask
Wood, 37.75 inches.
Bobo People
Burkina Faso
Collection of Dr. John Ross

Female Koba Antelope Mask
Polychrome wood, 21 inches.
Nuna people
Upper Volta River Basin, Burkina Faso
Ca. late 19th to early 20th century
Collection of Woods Davy

Monkey Mask
Polychrome wood, 13.5 inches.
Gurunsi (Nuna) People, Gnagna
Burkina Faso
Collection of Dr. John Ross

NIGERIA

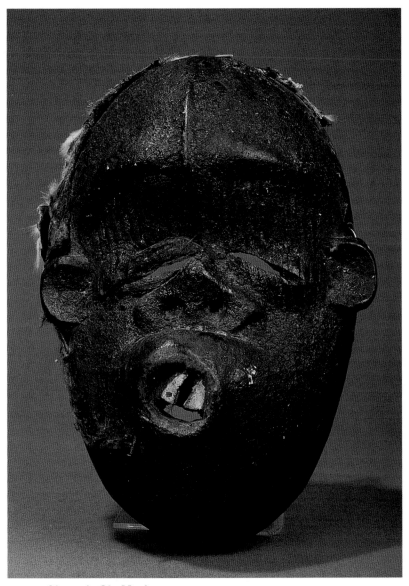

Okorosia Ojo Mask
Suppressor (*Omewuoha*). Polychrome
wood, animal skin, and hair, 9.5 inches.
Carved by Anozie
Igbo People
Mgbala Agwa, Nigeria
Ca. mid 20th century
Private Collection

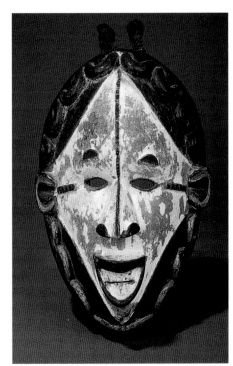

Okorosia Oma Mask
Leopard imitator. Polychrome
wood and fiber, 9.25 inches.
Igbo People
Mgbala Agwa, Nigeria
Ca. early to mid 20th century
Private Collection

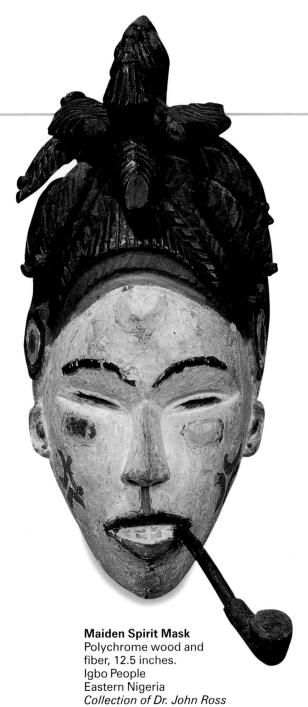

Maiden Spirit Mask
Polychrome wood and
fiber, 12.5 inches.
Igbo People
Eastern Nigeria
Collection of Dr. John Ross

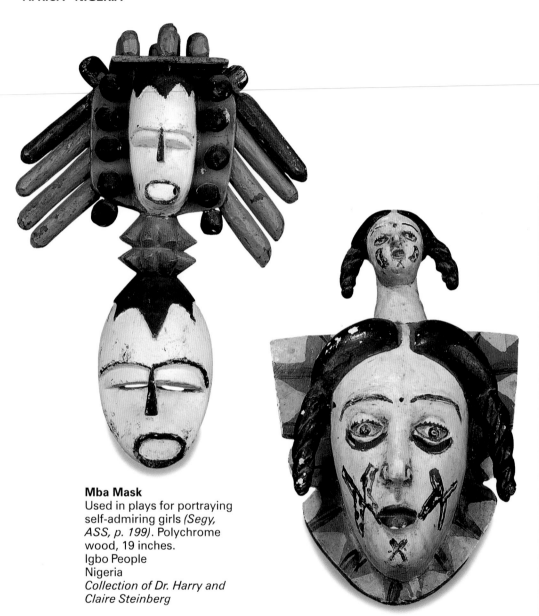

Mba Mask
Used in plays for portraying self-admiring girls *(Segy, ASS, p. 199)*. Polychrome wood, 19 inches.
Igbo People
Nigeria
Collection of Dr. Harry and Claire Steinberg

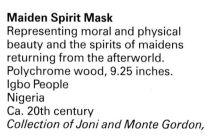

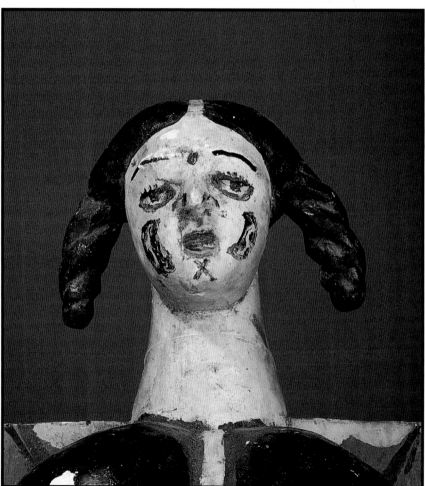

Maiden Spirit Mask
Representing moral and physical beauty and the spirits of maidens returning from the afterworld.
Polychrome wood, 9.25 inches.
Igbo People
Nigeria
Ca. 20th century
Collection of Joni and Monte Gordon,

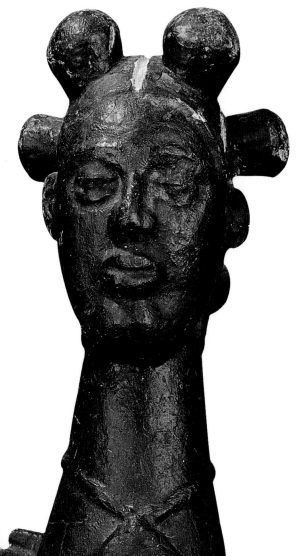

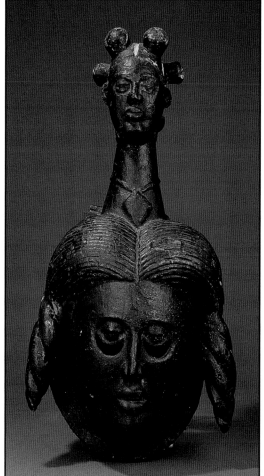

Face Mask
Female mask with second small head on
top. Polychrome wood, 22.25 inches.
Ibibio People
Eastern Nigeria
Collection of Dr. John Ross

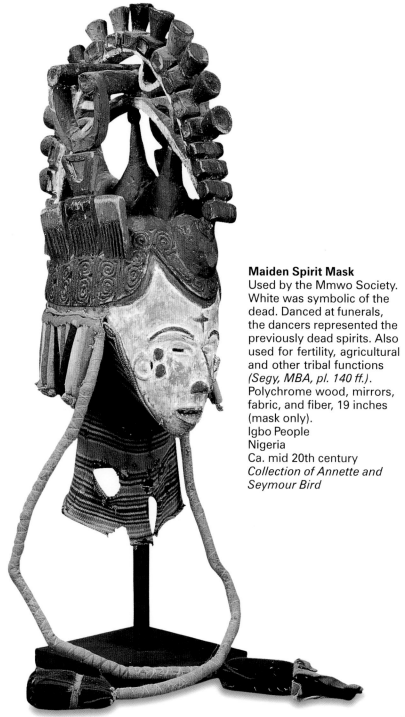

Maiden Spirit Mask
Used by the Mmwo Society.
White was symbolic of the
dead. Danced at funerals,
the dancers represented the
previously dead spirits. Also
used for fertility, agricultural
and other tribal functions
(Segy, MBA, pl. 140 ff.).
Polychrome wood, mirrors,
fabric, and fiber, 19 inches
(mask only).
Igbo People
Nigeria
Ca. mid 20th century
*Collection of Annette and
Seymour Bird*

43

I became enamored with African sculpture when first seeing some in galleries and museums. These sculptures have been influential in leading me to become a sculptor myself. Their spiritual quality is an endless source of inspiration.

Dr. Harry Steinberg

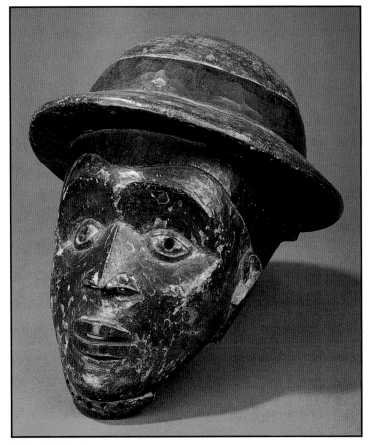

Colonial Mask
Because of the hat he wears, he is called "colonial." Polychrome wood, 13 inches.
Igbo People
Nigeria
Ca. early 20th century
Collection of Dr. Richard and Jan Baum

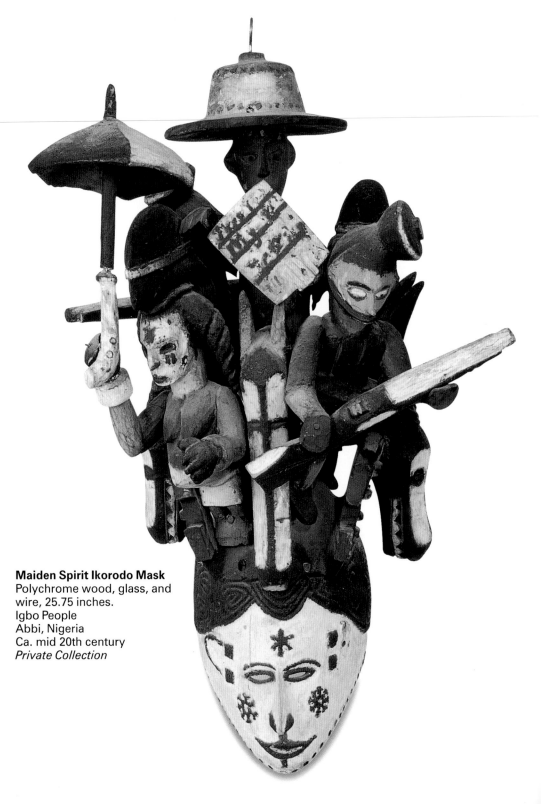

Maiden Spirit Ikorodo Mask
Polychrome wood, glass, and wire, 25.75 inches.
Igbo People
Abbi, Nigeria
Ca. mid 20th century
Private Collection

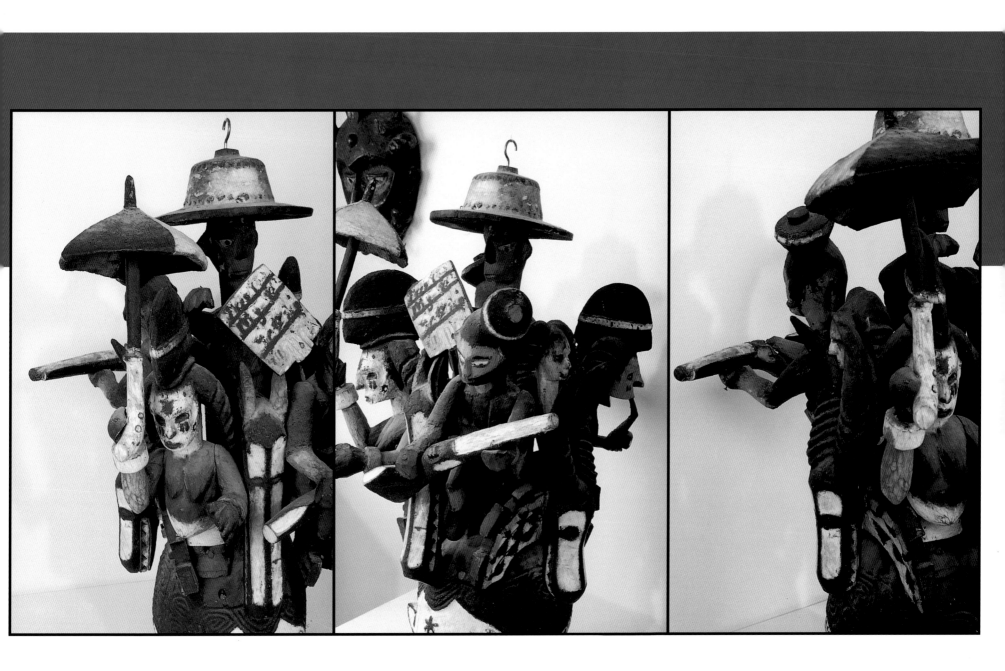

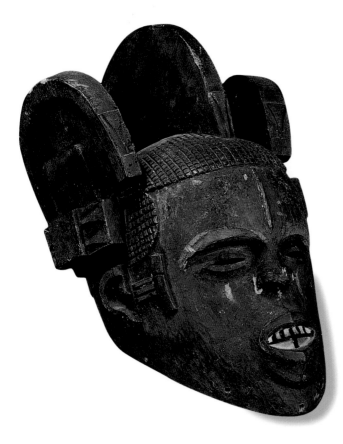

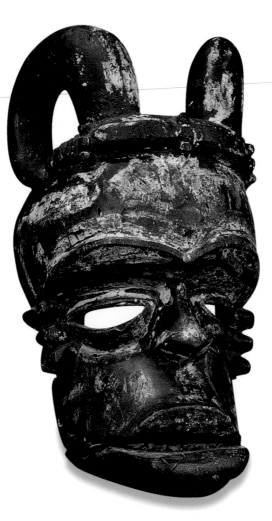

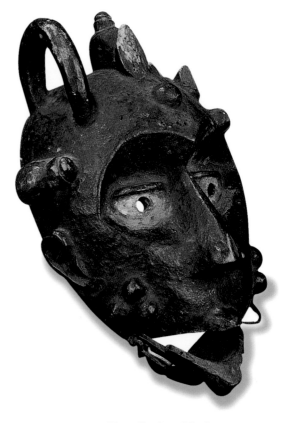

Maiden Helmet (Queen of Women)
Polychrome wood, 17 inches.
Igbo People
Eastern Nigeria
Collection of Dr. John Ross

Ekpo Society Mask
This black faced mask with horns and
articulated jaw is one of several used by
Ekpo Male Society members in their role
of honoring the dead and enforcing the
laws *(Segy, ASS, p. 199)*. Polychrome
wood and leather, 13.25 inches.
Anang Ibibio People
Eastern Nigeria
Collection of Dr. John Ross

Ekpo Society Mask
Polychrome wood and leather,
with articulated jaw, 11.5 inches.
Ibibio People
Eastern Nigeria
Collection of Dr. John Ross

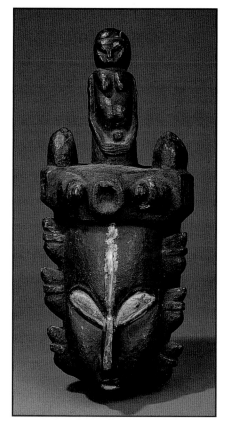

Ekpo Society Mask
Helps emphasize village autonomy to counterbalance centralized authority in the divine kingship at the court of Benin. Polychrome wood, 15.75 inches.
Bini People
Southwestern Nigeria
Ca. late 19th century
Collection of Woods Davy

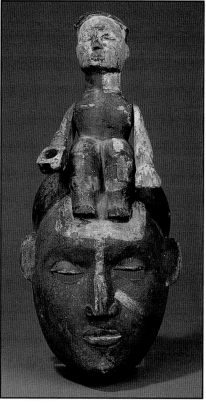

Face Mask
With male figure on superstructure. Polychrome wood, 16.75 inches.
Ibibio People
Eastern Nigeria
Collection of Dr. John Ross

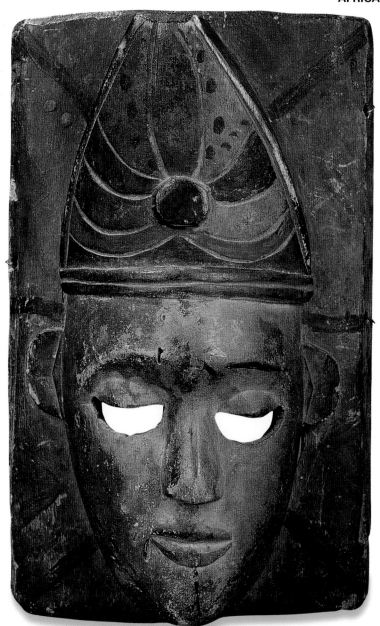

Bishop Mask
Bishop's face and miter has been incorporated into mask representing a symbol of religious authority.
Ibibio People
Eastern Nigeria
Collection of Dr. John Ross

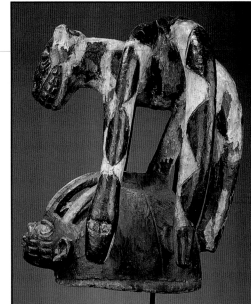

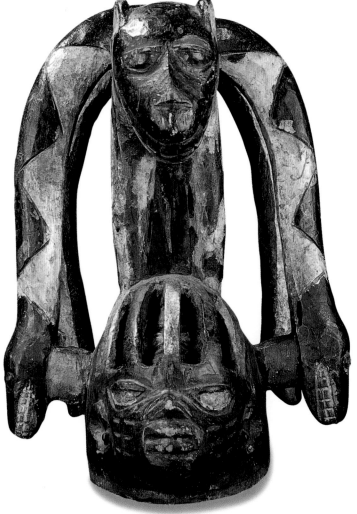

Gelede Mask
This mask is always danced in pairs and
honors the senior women in the Yoruba
society. The mask may take many stylistic
forms like the dramatic leopard and python
on this example. Polychrome wood, 18.5
inches.
Yoruba People
Nigeria
Ca. 2nd quarter 20th century
Collection of Diane and Ernie Wolfe III

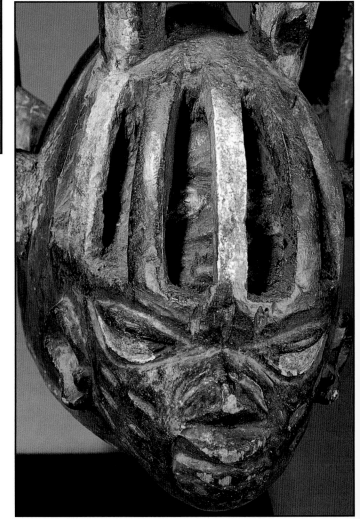

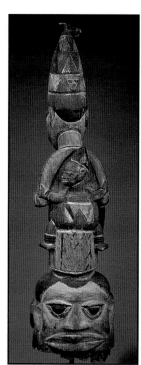

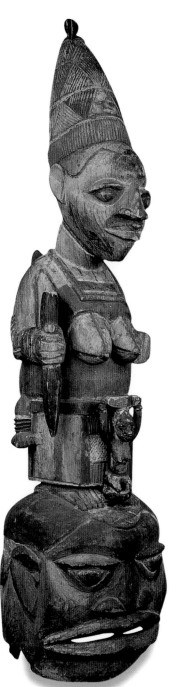

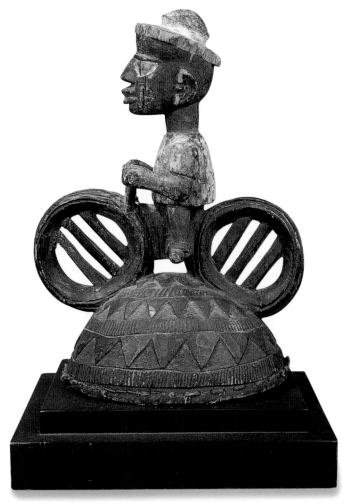

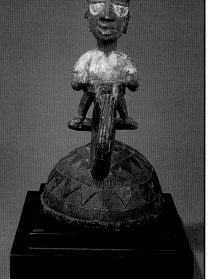

Egungun Mask
Male figure riding a bicycle. Poly-
chrome wood and fabric, 12.5 inches.
Yoruba People
Nigeria
Ca. early to mid 20th century
Collection of Suzan Lerer

Epa Mask
This mask honors the
mythical or cultural heroes
of the Yoruba. This ex-
ample is a matriarch
wearing a conical beaded
hat carrying a child,
surmounting the classic
Janus-form double faced
mask. Polychrome wood,
44 inches.
Yoruba People
Nigeria
Ca. early 20th century
*Collection of Diane and
Ernie Wolfe III*

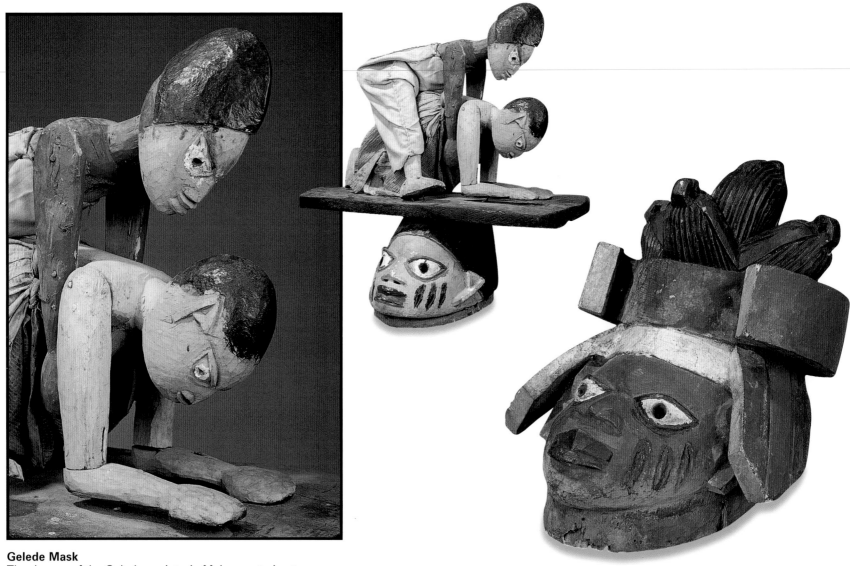

Gelede Mask
The dances of the Gelede society, in Meko, are trying to
placate the gods by providing entertainment for them (*Willett,*
p. 66). They are always colorful, and the top piece is often
humorous, as is this portrayal of a sexual act. Polychrome
wood and fabric, 19.75 inches.
Yoruba People
Nigeria
Ca. early to mid 20th century
Collection of Suzie Lerer

Plantain Marketing Woman Mask
The Gelede Society both honors and satirizes
the "mothers," danced in identical pairs by the
men. One of the roles satirized is that of the
market women. Polychrome wood, 16 inches.
Yoruba People
Anago, Pope, Nigeria
Ca. mid to late 20th century
Collection Ann and Monroe Morgan

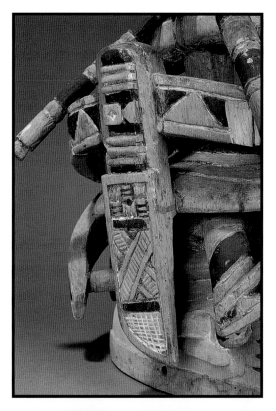

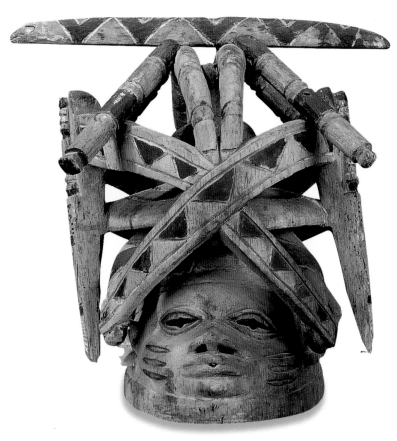

Gelede Mask
Polychrome wood, 14.25 inches.
Yoruba People
Nigeria
Collection of Dr. Harry and Claire Steinberg

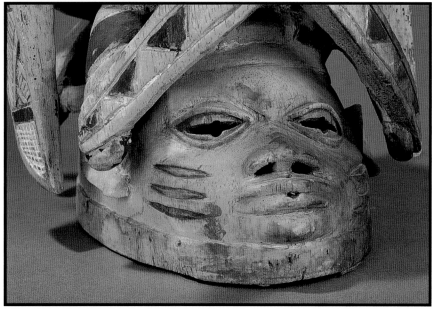

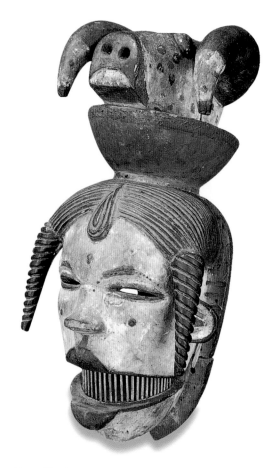

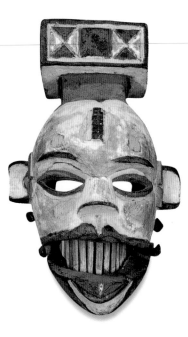

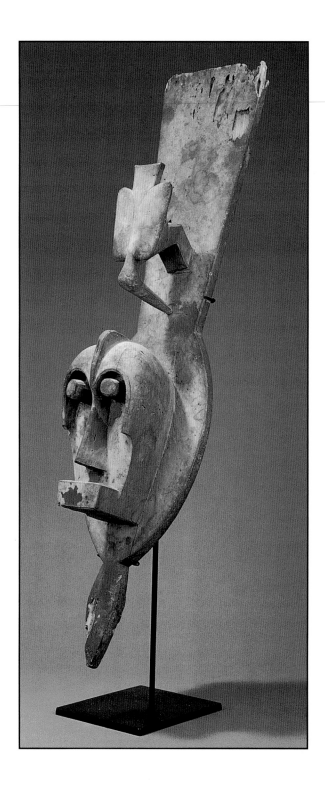

Above:
Face Mask
Articulated jaw. Polychrome wood, reed, and fiber, 9 inches with mouth open.
Ogoni People
Eastern Nigeria
Collection of Dr. John Ross

Right:
Water Spirit (Imole) Mask
The overall shape is that of a fish with projecting skull mounted by a bird. A form widespread among the river people, it represents the servant of Imole. It was worn horizontally on the hat so that as the wearer walked in the water it would appear to float *(Segy, ASS, p. 201).* Wood, 24 inches.
Ijaw People
Niger Delta Region, Southern Nigeria
Ca. mid 20th century
Collection of Woods Davy

Face Mask
This type of mask is also attributed to the Ekpo Society, where it was used by the Ibibio mutual aid officer *(Segy, MBA, pl. 134).* Articulated jaw. Polychrome wood, reed, and fiber, 13 inches.
Ogoni People
Nigeria
Ca. early 20th century
Collection of Dr. Richard and Jan Baum

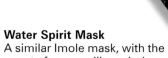

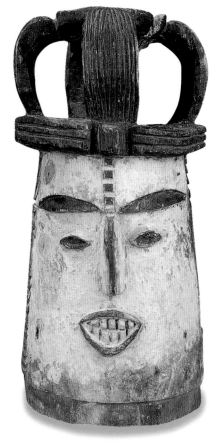

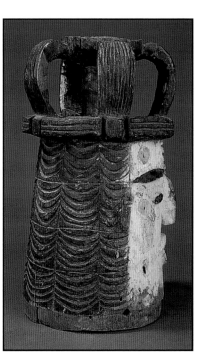

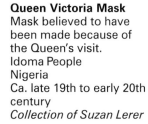

Water Spirit Mask
A similar Imole mask, with the snout of a crocodile and a human face. Polychrome wood, 26.75 inches.
Ijaw People
Niger Delta Region, Southern Nigeria
Ca. late 19th to early 20th century
Collection of Woods Davy

Queen Victoria Mask
Mask believed to have been made because of the Queen's visit.
Idoma People
Nigeria
Ca. late 19th to early 20th century
Collection of Suzan Lerer

Bush Cow Helmet Mask
Used by the Tsara Society in funeral ceremonies to lead the dead into the next world *(Segy, MBA, pl. 171)*. The mask places power and aggressive bush creatures at the service of human society and brings protection from non-human or supernatural forces in nature. Wood, 29 inches, front to back.
Chamba People
Benue River, Eastern Nigeria
Ca. early 20th century
Collection of Woods Davy

CAMEROON

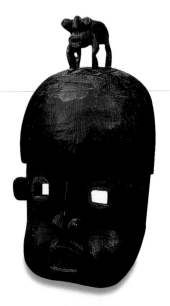

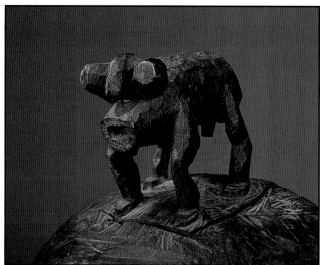

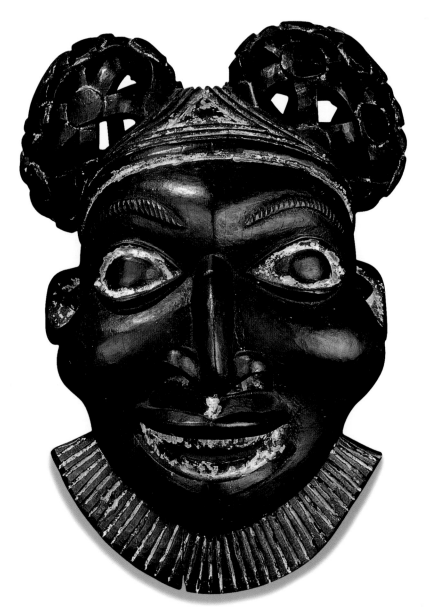

Left:
Bekom Helmet Mask
Expressing anthropomorphic bowing before the king and symbolic reproduction of social and political structure. Polychrome wood, 19 inches.
Cameroon
Ca. early to mid 20th century
Collection of Joni and Monte Gordon, Newspace, Los Angeles

Above:
Male Face Mask
Type used in the men's secret societies. Polychrome wood, 14.25 inches.
Widekum People
Western Forest lowlands, Cameroon
Ca. late 19th or early 20th century
Collection of Woods Davy

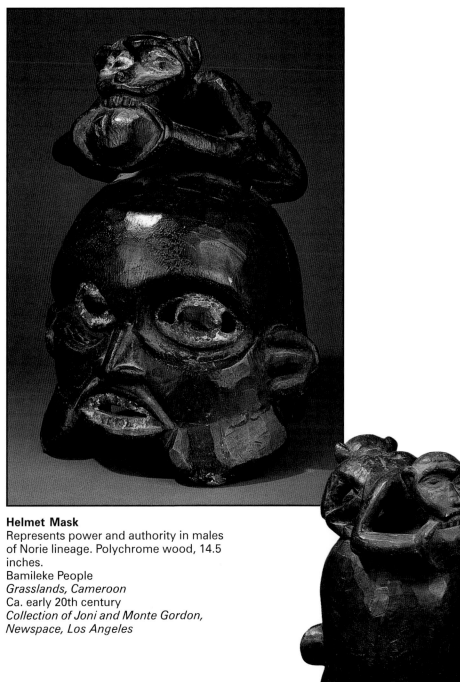

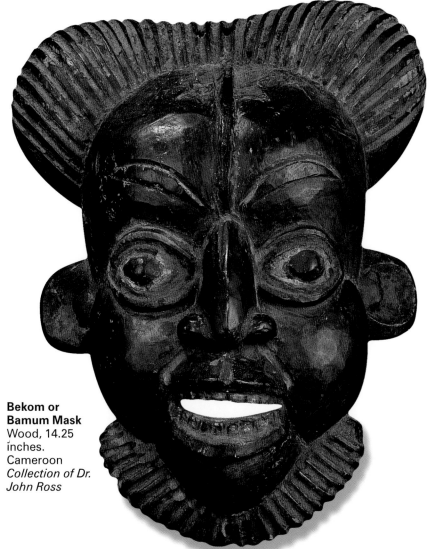

**Bekom or
Bamum Mask**
Wood, 14.25
inches.
Cameroon
*Collection of Dr.
John Ross*

Helmet Mask
Represents power and authority in males
of Norie lineage. Polychrome wood, 14.5
inches.
Bamileke People
Grasslands, Cameroon
Ca. early 20th century
*Collection of Joni and Monte Gordon,
Newspace, Los Angeles*

CONGO

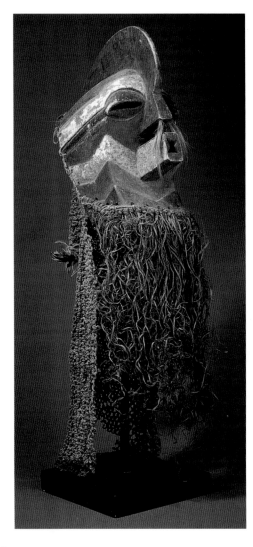

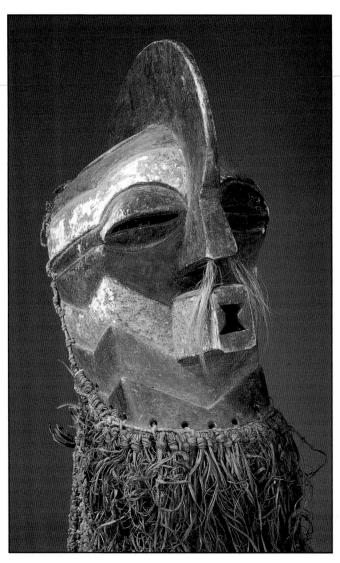

Kifwebe Association Mask
Exercises social control and seeks contributions, redistributing wealth. Also associated with cult of the dead. Wood, 15.5 inches.
Songye People
Democratic Republic of the Congo (Zaire)
Ca. mid 20th century
Collection of Joni and Monte Gordon, Newspace, Los Angeles

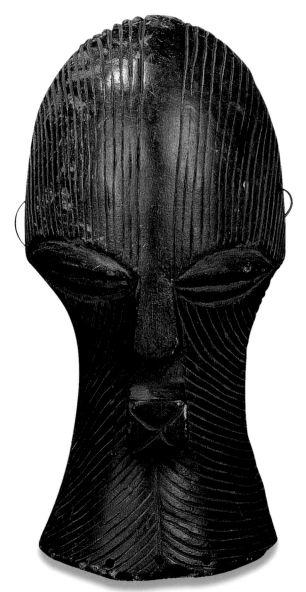

Male Kifwebe Mask
Masquerader of the Bwadi Bwa Kifwebe Society is feared as a supernatural creature, a malevolent and aggressive agent of authority that exercises social and political control for the ruling elite.
Polychrome wood and fiber, 34.75 inches.
Eastern Songye People
Kalunga Village, Kaseya Chiefdom, Democratic Republic of the Congo (Zaire)
Ca. mid 20th century
Collection of Woods Davy

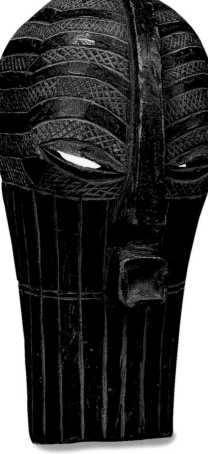

Female Kifwebe Hut Mask
Benevolent mask of protection
against disease and evil spirits.
Polychrome wood, 9 inches.
Eastern Songye People
Kabalo territory Democratic
Republic of the Congo (Zaire)
Ca. early to mid 20th century
Collection of Woods Davy

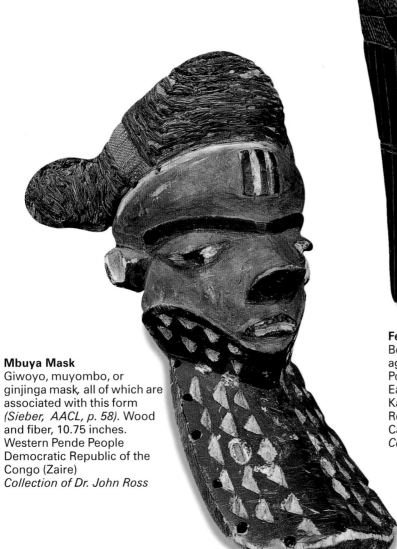

Mbuya Mask
Giwoyo, muyombo, or
ginjinga mask, all of which are
associated with this form
(Sieber, AACL, p. 58). Wood
and fiber, 10.75 inches.
Western Pende People
Democratic Republic of the
Congo (Zaire)
Collection of Dr. John Ross

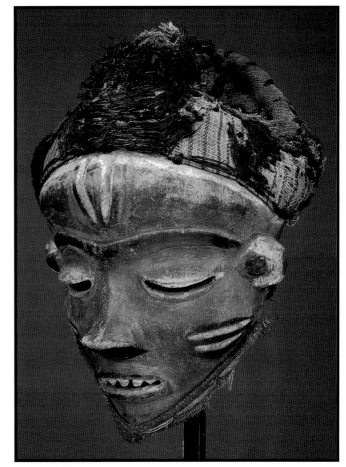

Mbuya Mask
Chief of clan. The Mbuya masks were worn by
boys as they returned to the village from their
circumcision rites and for various performances. Each mask had an identifiable personality *(Segy, ASS, p. 244).* Polychrome wood,
fabric, and fiber, 11.25 inches.
Western Pende People
Democratic Republic of the Congo (Zaire)
Collection of Dr. John Ross

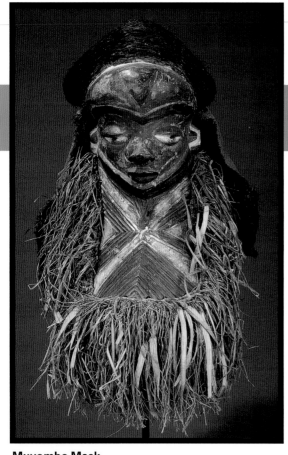

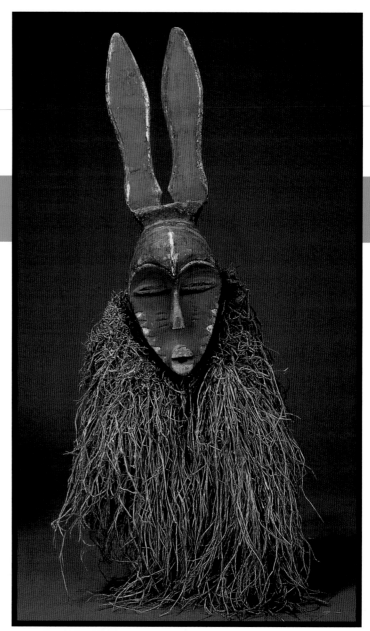

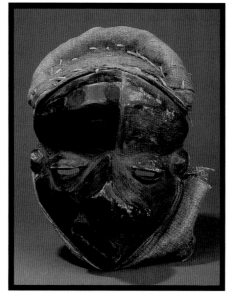

Muyombo Mask
The mask is associated with the dead. Polychrome wood, burlap, and fiber, 17 inches.
Western Pende (Kwango) People
Bandundu area, Democratic Republic of the Congo (Zaire)
Ca. mid 20th century
Collection of Woods Davy

Mboya Masi Mask
The clown, half-black and half-white. Distorted features refer to disease. Polychrome wood and fiber, 12 inches.
Pende People
Democratic Republic of the Congo (Zaire)
Collection of Joni and Monte Gordon, Newspace, Los Angeles

Mini Minyaangi Mask
Used in circumcision ceremonies. Polychrome wood and natural fibers, 22 inches.
Eastern Pende (Kasai) People
Democratic Republic of the Congo (Zaire)
Ca. early 20th century
Collection of Woods Davy

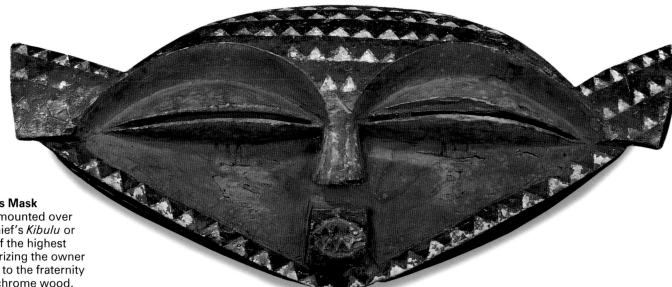

Top:
Panya Ngome, Chief's Mask
This mask was often mounted over the entrance of the chief's *Kibulu* or hut. It is the symbol of the highest order of chiefs, authorizing the owner to launch an initiation to the fraternity every ten years. Polychrome wood, 8.25 inches.
Eastern Pende (Kasai) People
Democratic Republic of the Congo (Zaire)
Ca. late 19th, early 20th century
Collection of Woods Davy

Left:
Soko-Mutu Mask
Mask associated with ancestors.
Wood, 9.75 inches.
Hemba People
Democratic Republic of the Congo (Zaire)
Ca. early 20th century
Collection of Joni and Monte Gordon, Newspace, Los Angeles

Right:
Hemba So'o Mask
Wood, 7.25 inches.
Hemba People
Shaba territory, Maniema area
Democratic Republic of the Congo (Zaire)
Ca. late 19th or early 20th century
Collection of Woods Davy

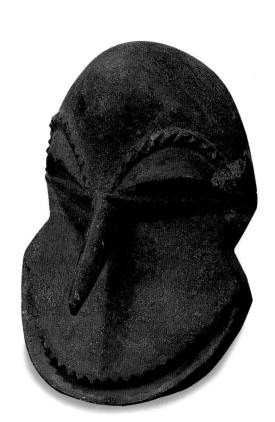

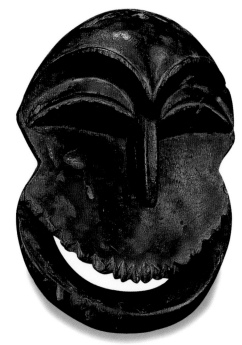

As an artist, I love the combination of aesthetic expression and magical power found in African art. For me, these tribal works have a mysterious purity that is almost addictive.

Woods Davy

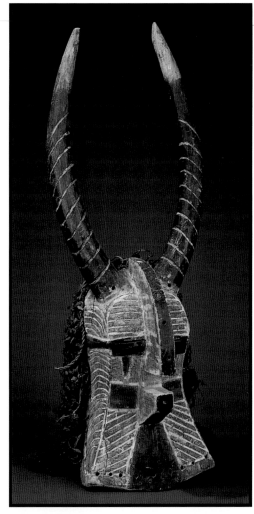

Kifwebe Mask
Female antelope mask. This is a masquerader who taught morals and social behavior based on character traits of certain animals.
Polychrome wood and fiber. 26.75 inches.
Luba People
Piana Bayo Chiefdom, Southeast of Ankoro, Democratic Republic of the Congo (Zaire)
Ca. mid 20th century
Collection of Woods Davy

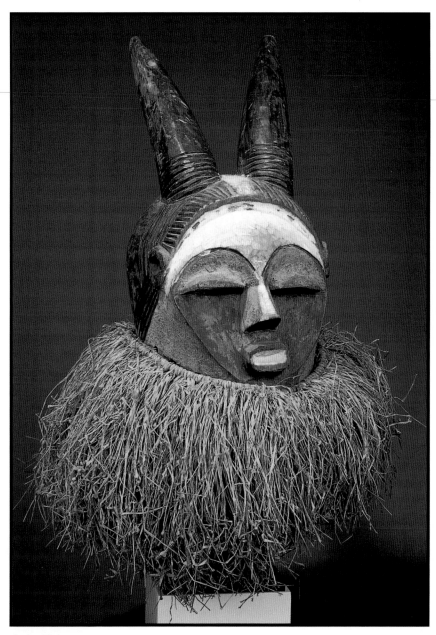

Suku Helmet
Polychrome wood and fiber, 28 inches overall.
Democratic Republic of Congo (Zaire)
Ca. 2nd Quarter 20th century
Collection of Dr. Richard and Jan Baum

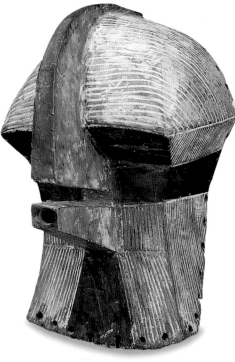

Male Kifwebe Mask.
Benevolent mask of protection, it also had the power to heal. Danced in new moon, funeral, and welcoming ceremonies and initiation rites.
Polychrome wood, 14.75 inches.
Luba People
Eastern Luba region, Democratic Republic of the Congo (Zaire)
Ca. early to mid 20th century
Collection of Woods Davy

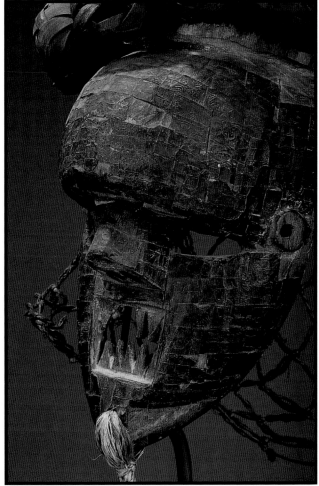

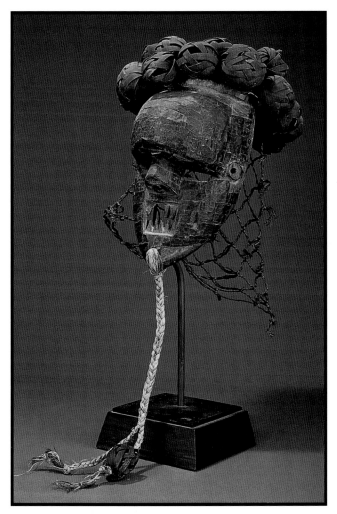

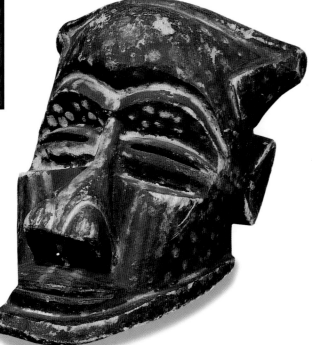

Left & above:
Mulandwa Mask of Mfuku Dance
The Salampusu are known as fierce warriors and
hunters, and their dances were integral to the building
of warlike ardor (*Huet, TDA, p. 156).* Wood, fiber, copper,
and skin, 12.5 inches (mask only).
Salampasu People
Luiza Region, Democratic Republic of the Congo (Zaire)
Ca. early to mid 20th century
Collection of Woods Davy

Right:
Mboom Helmet Mask
An initiation mask. Polychrome wood, 20 inches.
Kuba People
Democratic Republic of the Congo (Zaire)
Collection of Dr. John Ross

Fabric Mask
Male mask of the Ibangai Society.
30.5 inches overall.
Salampasu People
Democratic Republic of the Congo
(Zaire)
Ca. mid 20th century
*Collection of Shirley and David
Rowen*

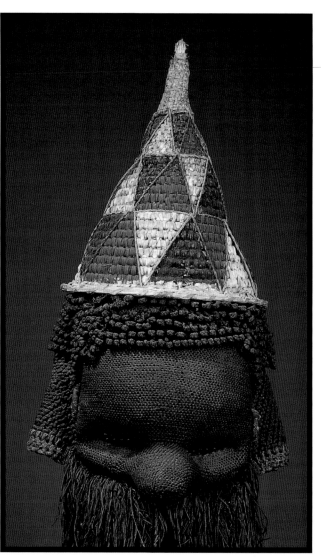

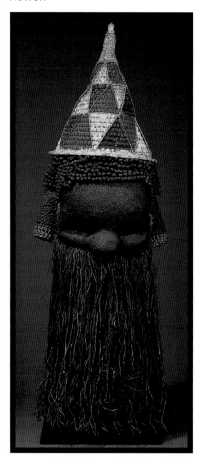

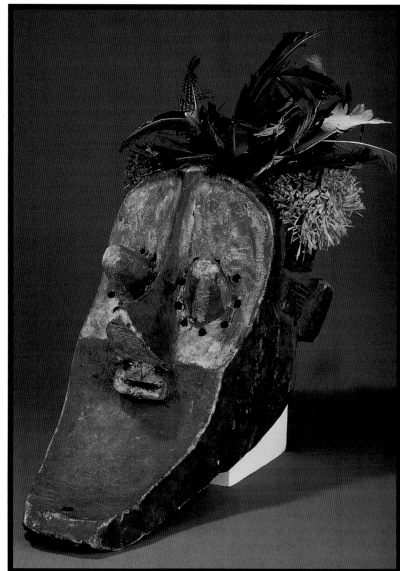

Circumcision Ceremonial Mask
Polychrome wood and natural materi-
als, 21 inches.
Kete People
Democratic Republic of the Congo
(Zaire)
Ca. mid 20th century
*Collection of Joni and Monte Gordon,
Newspace, Los Angeles*

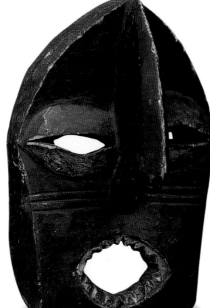

Hornbill Circumcision Mask
Mask for circumcision rite,
which was performed with bill of
hornbill bird. Wood, 13 inches.
Binji People
Mputu area, Democratic
Republic of the Congo (Zaire)
Ca. mid 20th century
Collection of Woods Davy

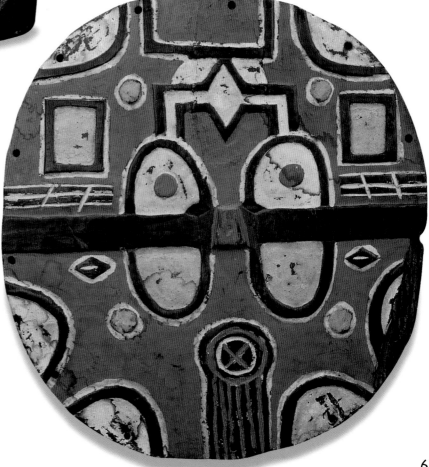

Polychrome Mask
Men's association mask
with abstract symbols that
express social and religious
group values. Polychrome
wood, 13.75 inches.
Teke People
Democratic Republic of the
Congo (Zaire)
Ca. mid 20th century
*Collection of Joni and
Monte Gordon, Newspace,
Los Angeles*

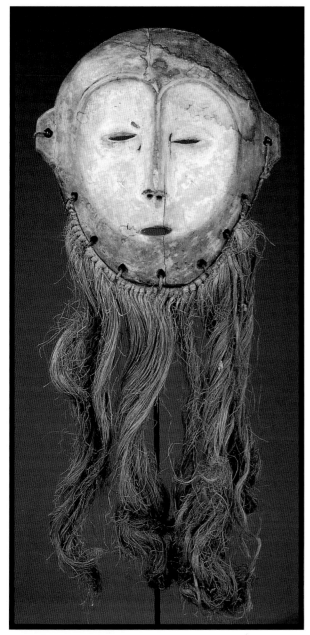

Bwami Society Mask
This mask is used by both men and woman as part of
the Bwami initiation ceremony. Often worn as pen-
dants rather than on the face. Wood and natural fibers,
23 inches.
Lega People
Democratic Republic of the Congo (Zaire)
Ca. early 20th century
Collection of Diane and Ernie Wolfe III

ANGOLA

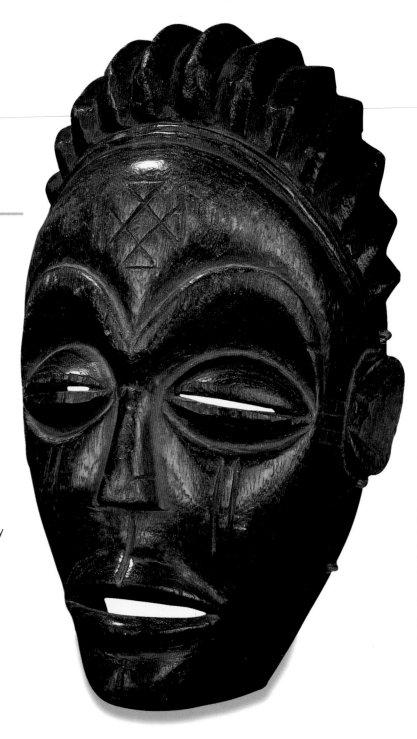

Mukanda Men's Initiation Mask
Known as *Mwana wa pwo,* this
mask symbolized the female
ancestor *(Segy, ASS, p. 270)* and
was used in male circumcision
ceremonies. The mask represents a
woman but is danced exclusively by
men. The scarification mark on the
forehead is called *cingelyengelye.*
Wood and fiber, 10 inches.
Chokwe People
Angola
Ca. early 20th century
*Collection of Diane and
Ernie Wolfe III*

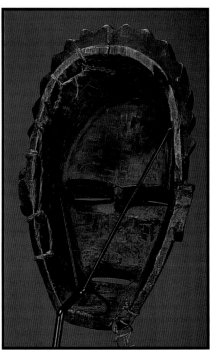

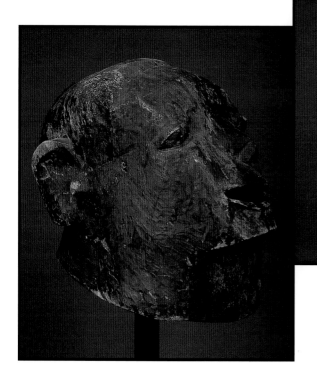

TANZANIA/MOZAMBIQUE

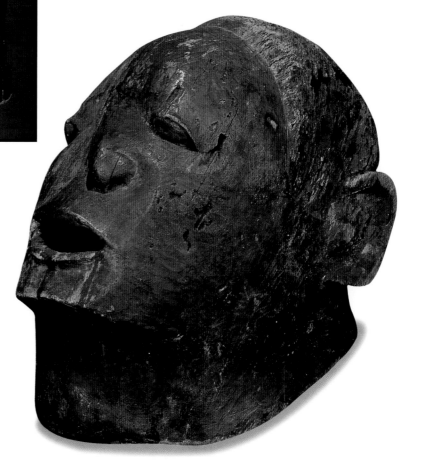

Helmet Mask
The Makonde migrated to eastern Africa from the southern Congo *(Willett, AA, pl. 14).* Segy relates their style to that of the Warega, southwest of Lake Victoria *(Segy, ASS, p. 271)* . These masks usually have carving on face which represents facial scarring. Wood and fiber, 11 inches.
Makonde People
Tanzania/Mozambique
Ca. early 20th century
Collection of Dr. Richard and Jan Baum

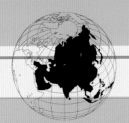

ASIA & *the Asian Pacific*

INDIA

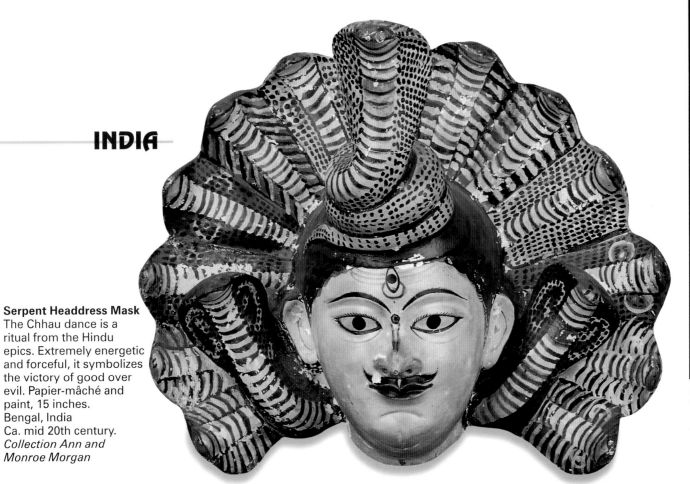

Serpent Headdress Mask
The Chhau dance is a ritual from the Hindu epics. Extremely energetic and forceful, it symbolizes the victory of good over evil. Papier-mâché and paint, 15 inches.
Bengal, India
Ca. mid 20th century.
Collection Ann and Monroe Morgan

7

9

Cloth Masks
Worn by animals in ceremonies. Cloth, mirrors, cowry shells, beads, and yarn.
Top: 13.5 inches; bottom: 10.5 inches.
India
Ca. late 20th century
Collection of Hope and Roy Turney

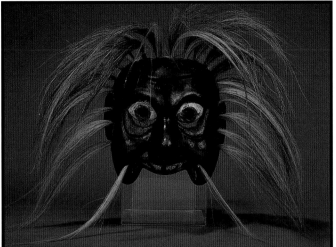

SRI LANKA

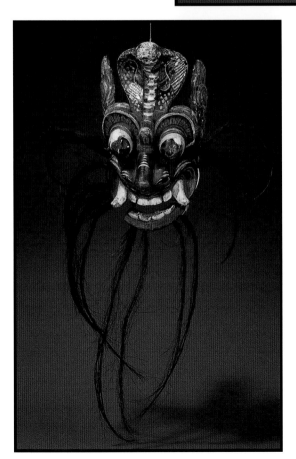

Above:
Half Mask
Polychrome wood, glass eyes, and hair, 5.75 inches.
Sri Lanka (Ceylon)
Ca. 20th century
Collection of Dr. John Ross

Left:
Kolam Sanniya Mask
Ceremonial mask for treating contagious disease, like cholera. The headdress contains the graphic form of a cobra. Polychrome wood and hair, 10 inches.
Sri Lanka (Ceylon)
Collection of Dr. John Ross

Right:
Kolam Mask
Polychrome wood, 7.25 inches.
Sri Lanka (Ceylon)
Ca. 20th century
Collection of Dr. John Ross

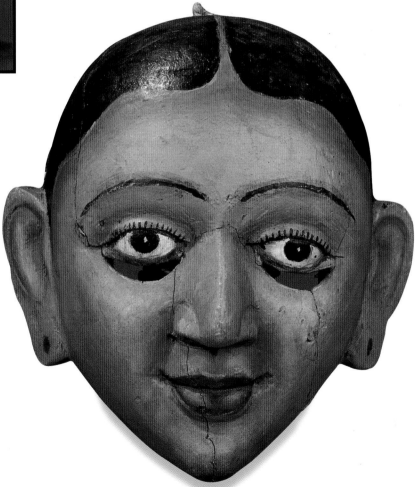

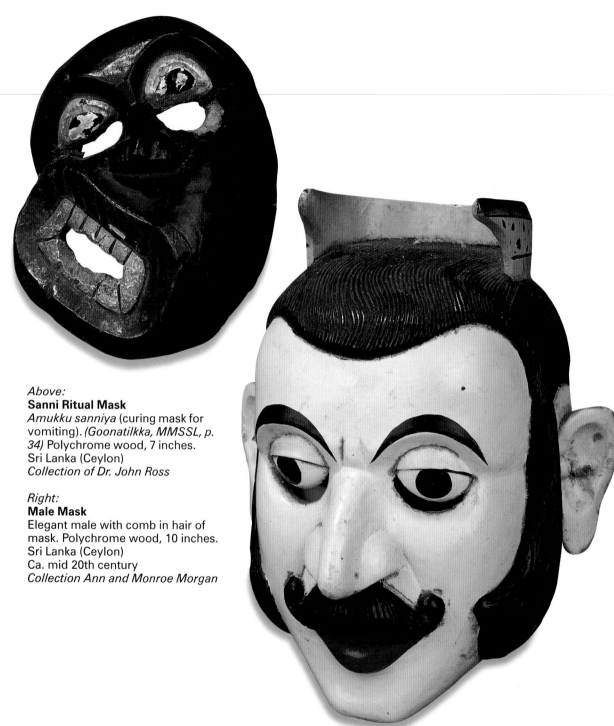

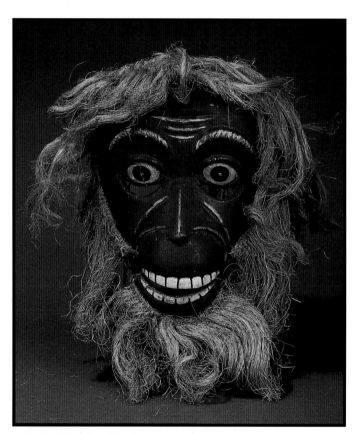

Above:
Sanni Ritual Mask
Amukku sanniya (curing mask for vomiting). *(Goonatilkka, MMSSL, p. 34)* Polychrome wood, 7 inches.
Sri Lanka (Ceylon)
Collection of Dr. John Ross

Right:
Male Mask
Elegant male with comb in hair of mask. Polychrome wood, 10 inches.
Sri Lanka (Ceylon)
Ca. mid 20th century
Collection Ann and Monroe Morgan

Kolam Monkey Mask
Polychrome wood and natural fiber, 10.5 inches.
Sri Lanka (Ceylon)
Collection of Dr. John Ross

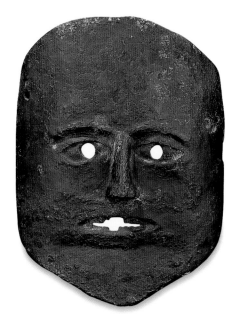

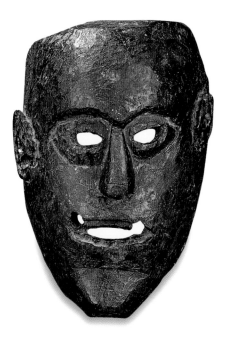

NEPAL

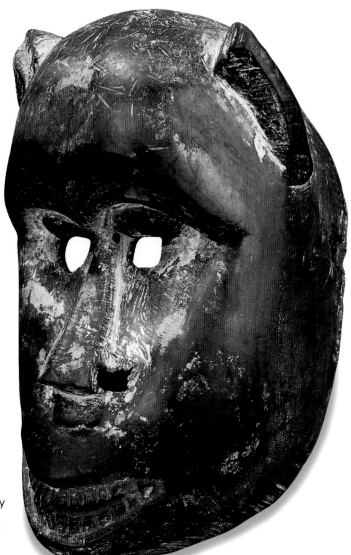

Face Mask
Polychrome wood, 10.5 inches.
Rai People
Middle Hills, Nepal
Ca. 18th to 19th century
Collection of Mayer and Faith Schames

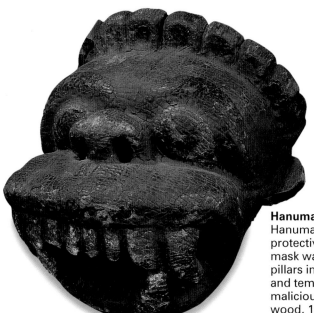

Shamanic Mask
Usually danced by village Shaman, the mask represents deities, ancestors or animals and is used to connect to local spirits on behalf of the village. Polychrome wood, 9.5 inches.
Gurung People
Middle Hills, Nepal
Ca. late 17th to early 18th century
Collection of Mayer and Faith Schames

Hanuman Mask
Hanuman is the monkey god, a protective deity. This large mask was suspended from pillars in houses, monasteries and temples to protect against malicious spirits. Polychrome wood, 18 inches.
Nepal
Ca. 17th to 18th century
Collection of Dorothy Wagle

Face Mask
Polychrome wood, 11.25 inches.
Terai, Nepal
Ca. late 18th to early 19th century
Collection of Mayer and Faith Schames

69

BHUTAN

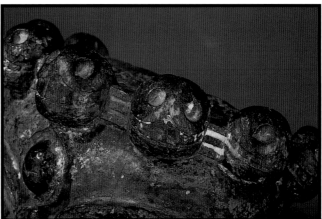

Temple Mask
Polychrome wood,
10.5 inches.
Bhutan
*Collection of Dr.
John Ross*

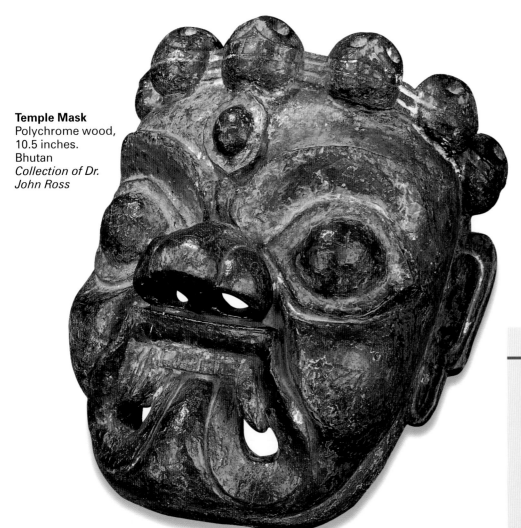

Our motivation for collecting has evolved over the years. Initially, we selected pieces which reflected the culture of the areas we were visiting and reminded us of our experiences there. Over time, we began to choose items for their intrinsic beauty, rarity, importance as ritual or cultural objects or for a special way materials were used or have aged – the patina of a bronze, a special sheen on a piece of wood, or an interesting combination of materials. Later we sought pieces which complement other objects we own to round out our collection. However, we always chose pieces which just spoke to us saying "take me home."

Jon and Cari Markell

TIBET

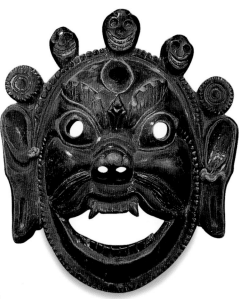

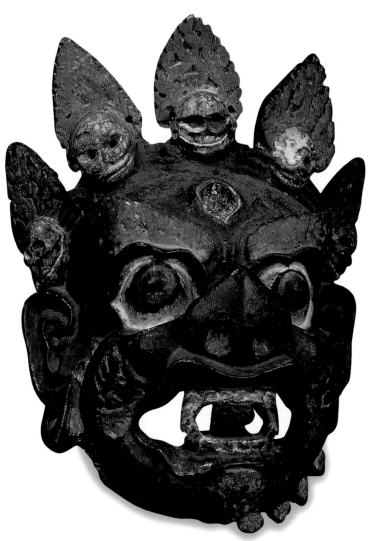

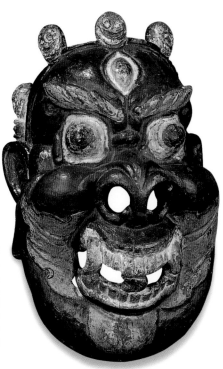

Gompo Mask
Buddhist protector. Polychrome
wood, 10.5 inches.
Tibet
Collection of Dr. John Ross

Gompo Mask
Protective deity. Polychrome
wood, 14 inches.
Tibet
Ca. 18th century
*Collection of Jerry Solomon,
Los Angeles*

Gompo Mask
Protection deity.
Polychrome wood,
14.5 inches.
Tibet
Ca. 18th century
*Collection of Jerry
Solomon, Los Angeles*

Gompo Mask
Protective deity. Polychrome
wood, 11.75 inches.
Tibet
Ca. 17th century
*Collection of Jerry Solomon,
Los Angeles*

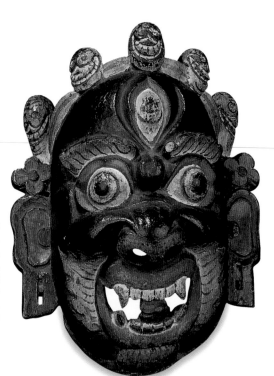

Gompo Mask
Buddhist protector.
Polychrome wood,
13.5 inches.
Tibet
Ca. 20th century
*Collection of Dr.
John Ross*

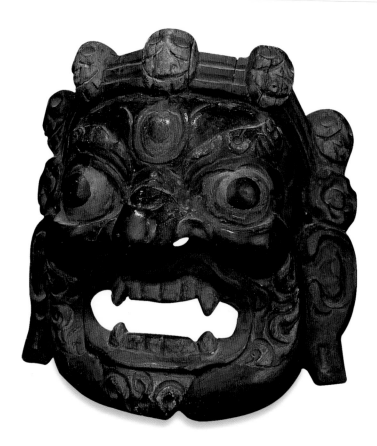

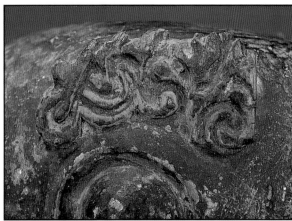

Temple Mask
Animal form, possibly a lion.
Polychrome wood, 10.25 inches.
Tibet
Collection of Dr. John Ross

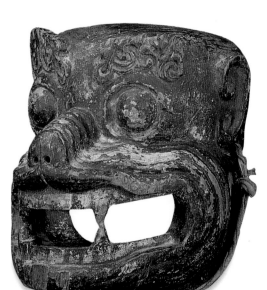

Bhairava or Mahakala Mask
The iconography is believed to be correct
for either Bhairava, the fierce terrific form
of the Hindu God Shiva, or Mahakala, the
tantric god of Buddhism and defender of
law. Polychrome wood, 9.5 inches.
Nepal or possibly Tibet
Ca. 2nd quarter 20th century
Collection of Jon and Cari Markell

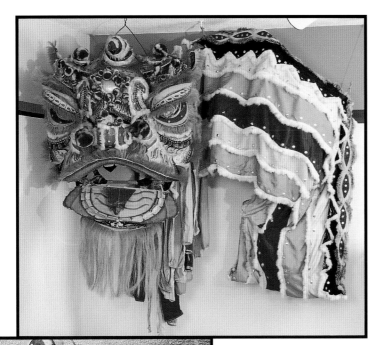

CHINA

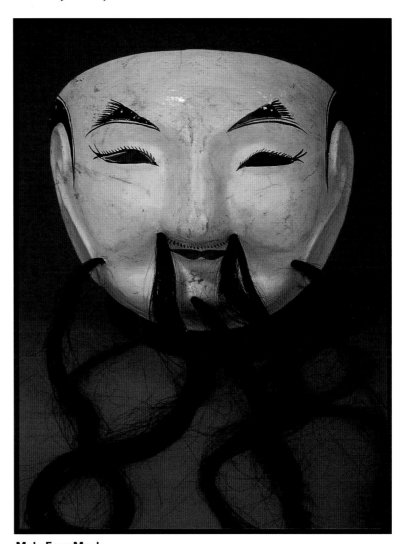

Blessing Lion
Danced for the past 30-40 years in China Town, Los Angeles, California. The yellow lion (symbolizing wisdom of old age) blesses businesses, appears in funerals, weddings and birthdays. Battery-powered eyes light up, and the eyelids and jaw are movable. Papier-mâché, glass, bristles, synthetic fur, fabric, and paint. The head is 30 inches tall with the mouth closed.
Fatson Village near Canton China
Ca. mid 20th century
Collection of Jim and Jeanne Pieper

Male Face Mask
Papier-mâché with wood bar inside the mask used as grip for the teeth of the mask wearer. 6.75 inches.
China
Ca. mid 20th century
Collection Ann and Monroe Morgan

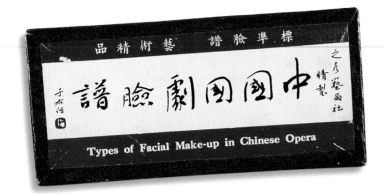

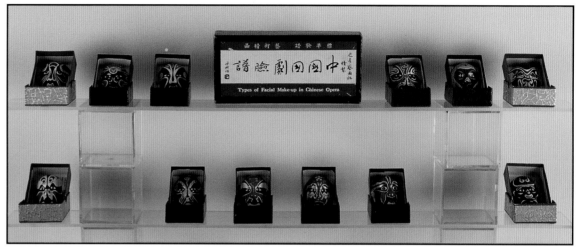

Chinese Face Painting Masks
These masks are used as guides for painting the face in traditional Chinese theater. Originally the face painting was designed to scare the enemy when one was going into battle. 2.5 inches.
China
Ca. late 20th century
Collection Marlan Clarke

Left to right:
Ching-wu Chu. Prince who founded the Ching Dynasty by defeating the Sung and in turn was defeated by Genghis Kahn.

Yang Chi. A member of the army who guards treasure, then joins the underground army when the treasure is stolen.

Yu-ch'ih Pao Lin. A young general who was raised by his father's enemy, rejoins his real father and defeats his foster father.

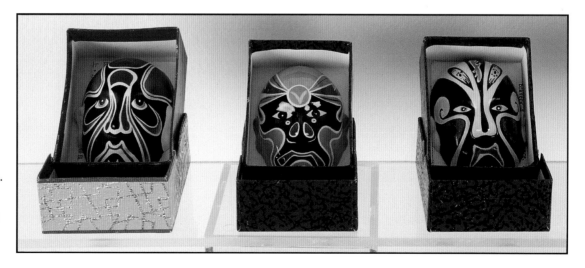

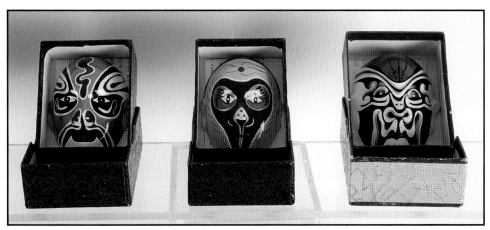

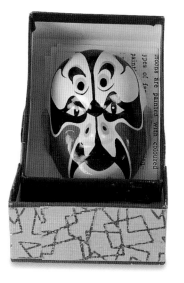

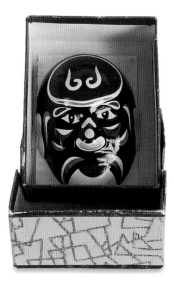

Left to right:

Kai Lu Wen. Korean General (608-914 AD) who possessed magical powers. Indicated by the mark on his forehead.

Monkey King. Raises havoc in Heaven

Zhou T'Sang. A brave and honest general who becomes one of three assistants to the war god and posseses magical powers.

Zhang Fei. One of the top five generals from the state of Shu during the three kingdoms. Heavy drinker, indicated by his pink color.

Pa'n Kuan. An official from the nether world. He officiates the book of deeds and is met upon death.

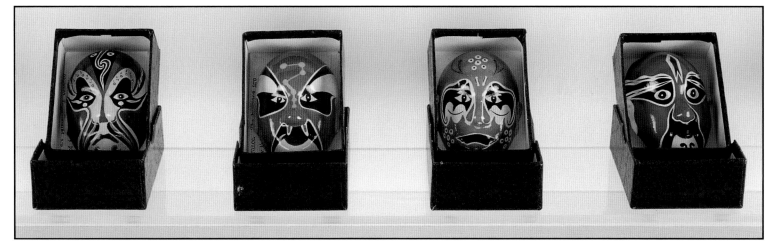

Left to right:

Chin Mein Hu. This means "green faced tiger," a mystical character who was a bandit and could carry off women.

Three Tile Big Dipper. The constellation pattern on his forehead and the universal side of the gods.

Deer Boy. An assistant to the gods, who looks after all magical plants in the garden. He symbolizes prosperity.

Sho'Ch'ao. A general whose blue color stands for bravery. The mark on his forehead means he carries a spear.

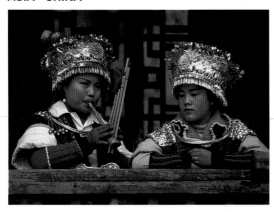

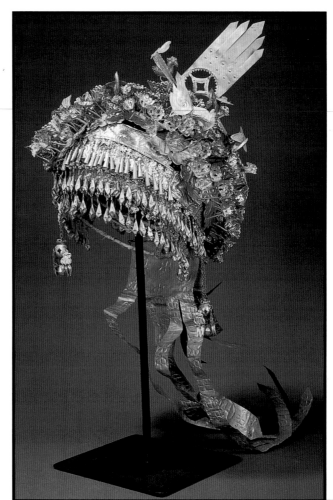

Silver Headdress
Guizou Province, South
West China
Ca. late 20th century
*Photos: Shirley and
David Rowen*

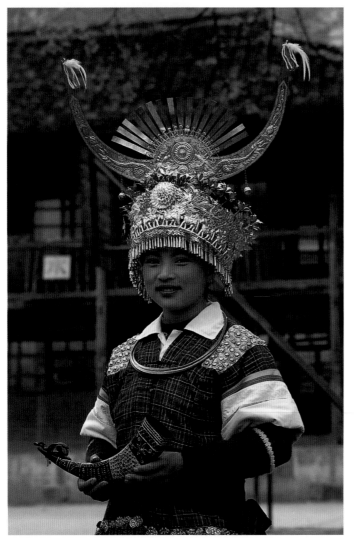

Silver Headdress
Metal, 12.5 inches in
diameter.
Guizou Province, South
West China
Ca. late 20th century
*Collection of Shirley and
David Rowen*

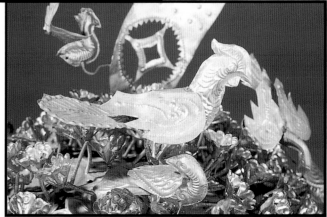

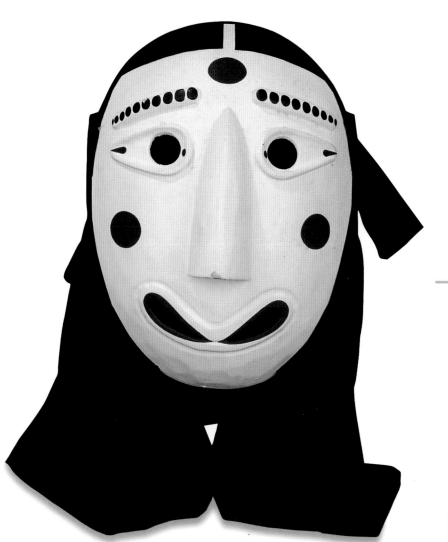

KOREA

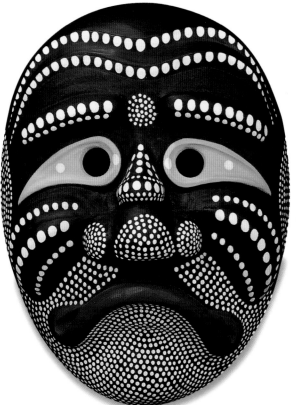

Above:
Woman "Waejanghyo" (Procuress) Mask
The play is Pyol Nori, a series of community folk dances. Most of the themes are satires on the upper class of society and the clergy. Polychrome wood and cloth, 9.5 inches.
Korea
Ca. late 20th century
Collection of Ann and Monroe Morgan

Right:
Theater Mask
Possibly representing Nojang (the old Priest) in the Bongsan or Kangryong, or Chwi Bali (Prodigal) in the Kangryong *(Song, MSUT, pl. 26 & 39)*. Polychrome wood and cloth, 9.75 inches.
Korea
Late 20th century
Collection of Marlan Clarke

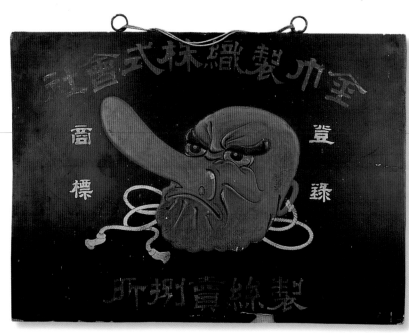

Trade Sign
Black lacquer wood sign with image of Tengu. Sign believed to advertise a dry goods store and "Tengu," the brand name for a thread. Polychrome wood, 15 x 21.5 inches.
Japan
Ca. late 19th to early 20th century.
Collection of Ann and Monroe Morgan

JAPAN

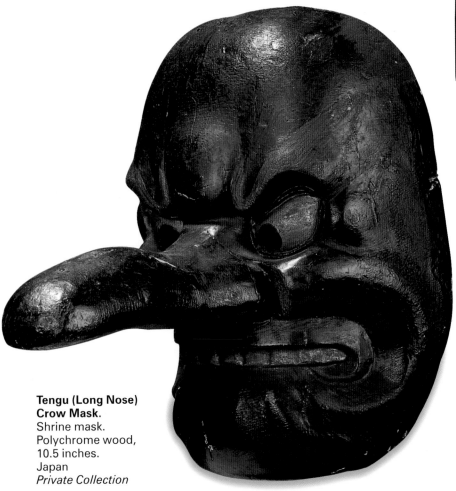

Tengu Mask
Represents playful forest demon. Polychrome wood and fiber, 6.5 inches.
Japan
Collection of Dr. John Ross

Tengu (Long Nose) Crow Mask.
Shrine mask.
Polychrome wood, 10.5 inches.
Japan
Private Collection

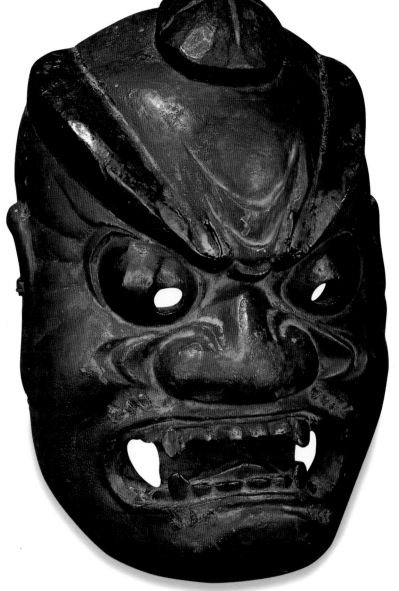

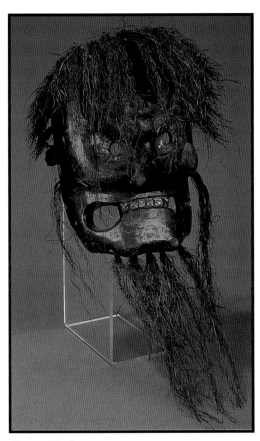

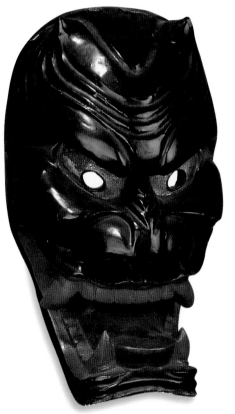

Tengu Mask
Represents a playful demon dwelling in the forest. Masks are used in rural village Shinto festivals and processions. Polychrome wood and fiber, 7 inches (head only).
Japan
Ca. mid 19th century
Collection of Ann and Monroe Morgan

Tengu Shrine Mask
Deals with donations to the shrine.
Polychrome wood, 10.5 inches.
Japan
Ca. late 17th to early 18th century
Private Collection

Ryu Oni Shrine Mask
Devil type mask. Wood and lacquer, 11.75 inches.
Japan
Private Collection

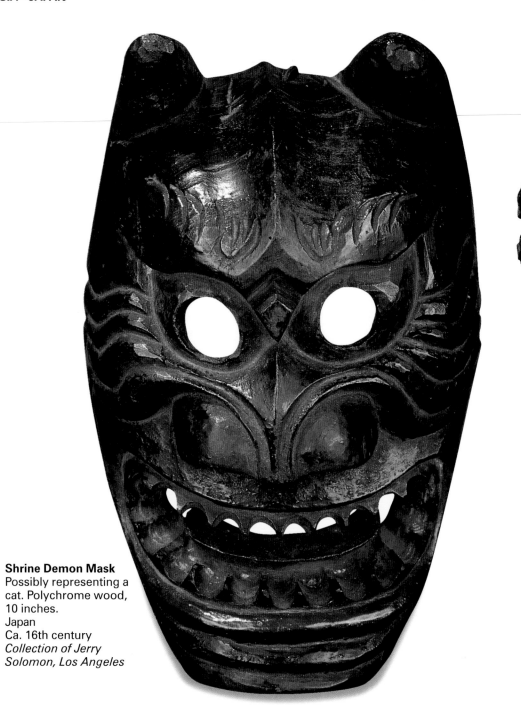

Ryu Oni or Dragon Demon Mask
Wood, 12.25 inches.
Saiga City, Japan
Ca. 16th century
*Collection of Jerry Solomon,
Los Angeles*

Shrine Demon Mask
Possibly representing a
cat. Polychrome wood,
10 inches.
Japan
Ca. 16th century
*Collection of Jerry
Solomon, Los Angeles*

Demon Shrine Mask
Open mouthed and
fanged shrine mask.
Wood, 9.25 inches.
Japan
*Collection of Jerry
Solomon, Los Angeles*

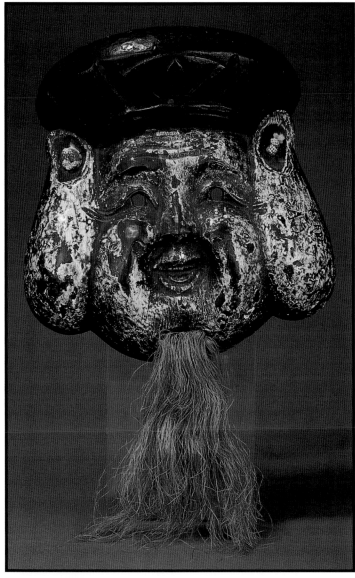

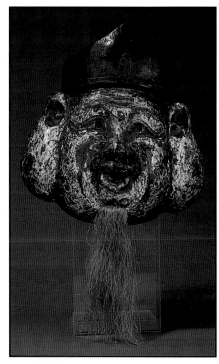

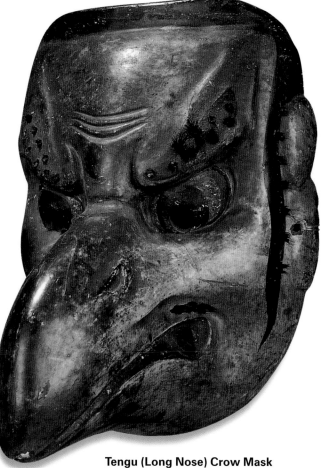

Daikoku Mask
Paired with Ebisu. One of the seven happy gods, this is the god of the wealth of the earth. Often used in Kyogen dramas. *(Bushell, NM, p. 114).* Polychrome wood and fiber, 8.5 inches.
Japan
Ca. late 16th to early 17th century
Collection of Jerry Solomon, Los Angeles

Ebisu Mask
Paired with Daikoku mask, this god of the wealth of the sea is another of the seven happy gods. Often used in Kyogen dramas. *(Bushell, NM, p. 114).* Polychrome wood and fiber, 9 inches.
Japan
Ca. late 16th to early 17th century
Collection of Jerry Solomon, Los Angeles

Tengu (Long Nose) Crow Mask
As part of Japanese folk dance, these tengu masks often represent goblins *(Bushell, NM, p. 109).* Polychrome wood and hair, 8 inches.
Japan
Private Collection

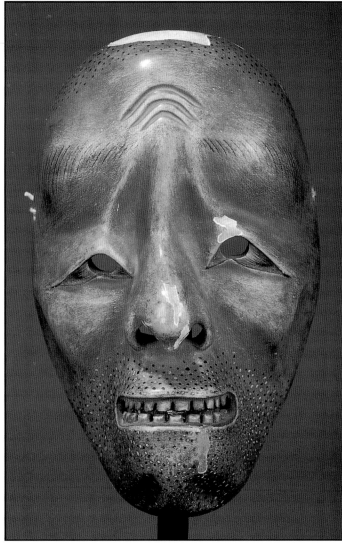

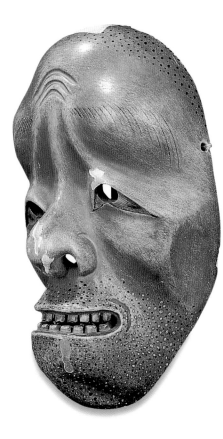

Kyogen Mask
Folk mask very finely carved from hardwood.
Polychrome wood, 8 inches.
Japan
Collection: of Dr. John Ross

Me No Shita Ho Face Protector
Armor mask covering the nose and throat worn
by the Samurai. Enameled metal and natural
bristles, 8 inches.
Japan
Ca. Edo period (1615-1867 AD)
Collection of Dr. John Ross

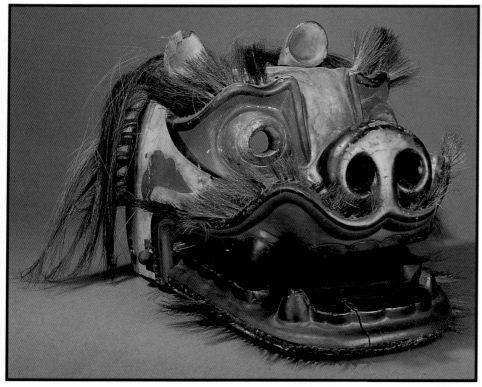

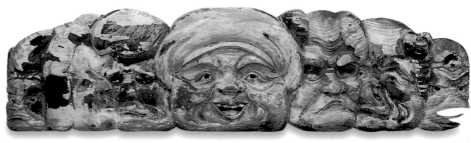

Sign
Believed to be an old mask maker's sign. Polychrome wood, 9.25 inches high, 36 inches wide.
Japan
Private Collection

Above:
Shi Shi
Lion mask. The *shishimai* or lion dance is found throughout Asia, and is often associated with New Years celebrations *(Mack, MAAE, p. 138).* Polychrome wood and hair, with a hinged mouth, 5 inches front to back.
Japan
Collection of Ann and Monroe Morgan

Right:
Child's Shi Shi Mask
Polychrome wood with metal hinges, 5 inches.
Tokyo, Japan
Ca. mid 19th century
Collection of Jim and Jeanne Pieper

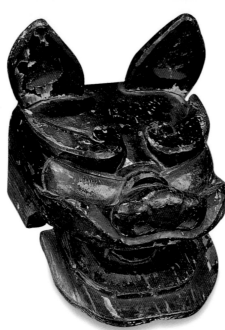

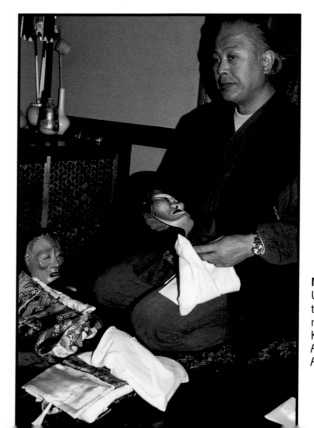

Mask Maker
Unwrapping treasured masks.
Kyoto, Japan
Photo: Jim Pieper

83

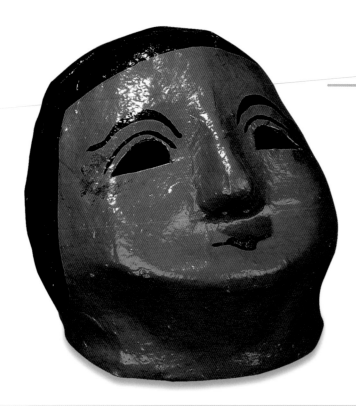

SINGAPORE

Female Big Head Mask
Frequently dances with the lion in Chinese celebrations. Papier-mâché, 9.25 inches. Singapore
Ca. late 20th century
Collection of Jim and Jeanne Pieper

INDONESIA

If we knew why we collect, it would lose its magic to us. Collecting satisfies deep urges for search and rescue, inquiry and experiences. Collecting for us is being fully alert to content, exotic regions, bewildering human expressions, rituals and materials in order to find meaning from remote people and countries. We enjoy tracing objects back to their human connections while accepting that we may never fully know their use and context. Collecting is a wild ride emphasizing the small space between birth and death.

Joni and Monte Gordon

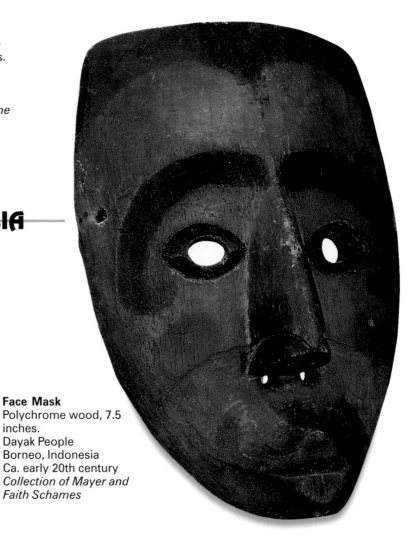

Face Mask
Polychrome wood, 7.5 inches.
Dayak People
Borneo, Indonesia
Ca. early 20th century
Collection of Mayer and Faith Schames

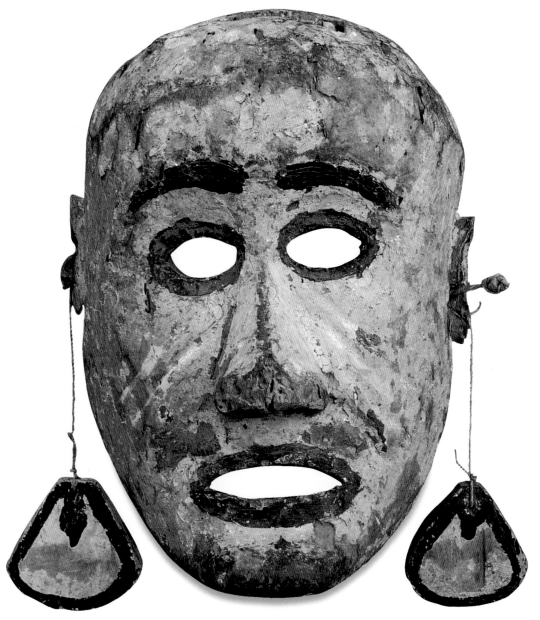

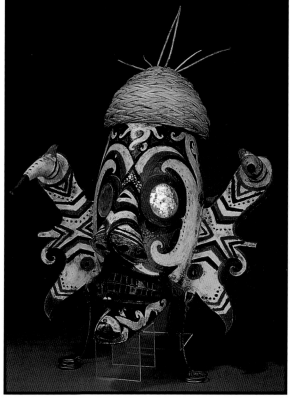

Hudog Mask
Wood, twine, hair, mirror, woven hat, and metal, 17.75 inches.
Kayan People
Central Borneo, Indonesia
Ca. 20th century
Collection of Jerry Solomon, Los Angeles

Rice Festival Mask
Polychrome wood and fiber, 10.25 inches.
Iban, Dayak People
Enicari River, Sarawak, Borneo
Collection of Dr. John Ross

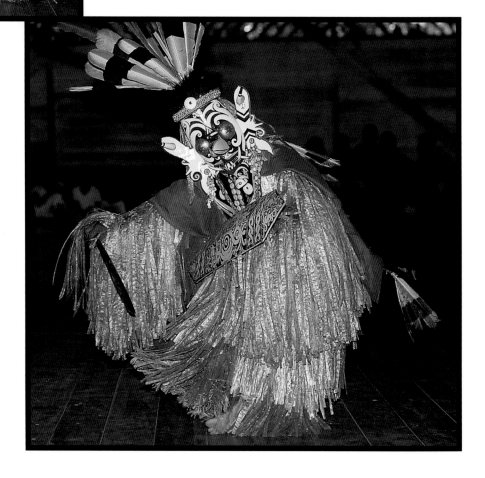

Hudog Mask
Datah Bilane Village,
Borneo, Indonesia
*Photo: Shirley and David
Rowen*

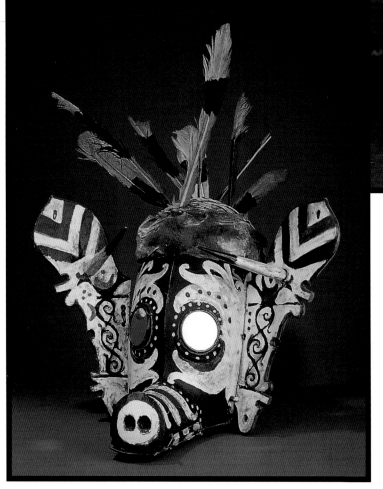

Hudog Mask
Worn in performances connected with agricultural ceremonies,
especially a wild boar hunt. Thought to represent ancestors
and also used in mortuary ceremonies. Polychrome wood,
feathers, basketry, mirror, and fur, 18 inches (head only).
Dayak people
Borneo, Indonesia
Ca. mid 20th century
Collection of Ann and Monroe Morgan

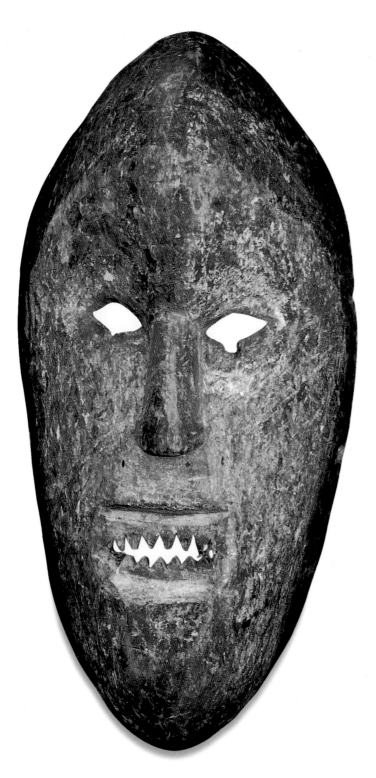

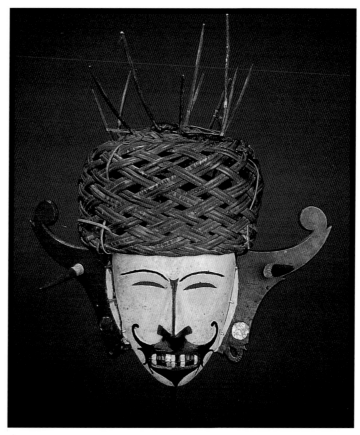

Above:
Kenyak-Kayan Mask
Javanese influence. Polychrome wood, basketry, fiber, and metal, 10.5 inches overall.
Dayak People
East Kalimantan, Borneo, Indonesia
Ca. 20th century
Collection of Jerry Solomon, Los Angeles

Left:
Long House Mask
Hung in long house to separate a section used by a single person and also used to ward off evil spirits. Polychrome wood, 19.5 inches.
Dayak People
Second Division River System, Borneo
Collection of Dr. John Ross

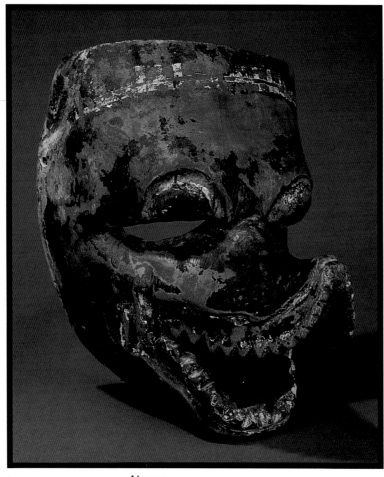

Above:
Topeng Aso
This mask represents a protective beast.
Described as a dog or a dragon, it might appear
as a symbol on a baby carriage, building, doors,
medicine bottles, or even coffins. Polychrome
wood, 7.75 inches.
Kalimantan, Indonesia
Ca. 1975
Collection of Jon and Cari Markell

Right:
Monkey Mask
Polychrome wood, 8.75 inches.
Island of Kalimantan, Borneo, Indonesia
Collected in early 1980s
Collection of Mr. and Mrs. David E. Hayen

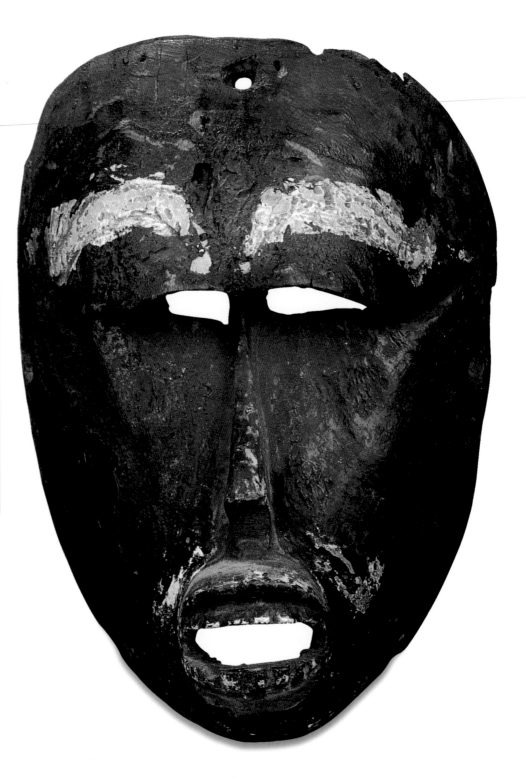

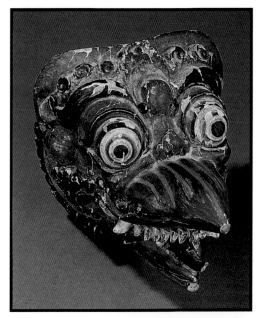

Topeng Jatayu
The brave bird who in the epic Ramayana tries to rescue the kidnapped wife of the King Rama and is mortally wounded, but tells Rama of the abduction. Polychrome wood, 6 inches.
Bali, Indonesia
Ca. mid 20th century
Collection of Jon and Cari Markell

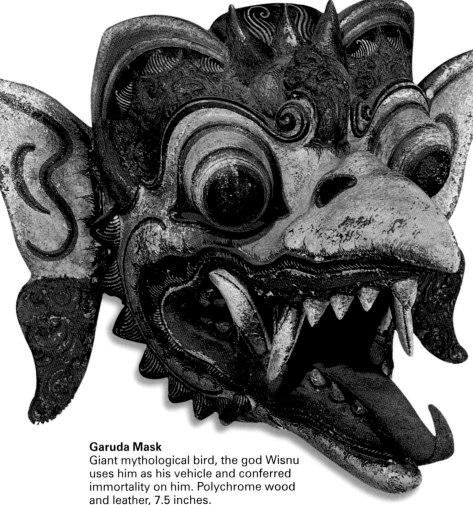

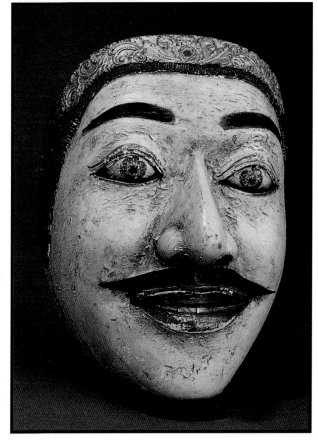

Garuda Mask
Giant mythological bird, the god Wisnu uses him as his vehicle and conferred immortality on him. Polychrome wood and leather, 7.5 inches.
Bali, Indonesia
Ca. 3rd quarter 20th century
Collection of Jim and Jeanne Pieper

Topeng Dalem
This is a prototypical Balinese king. Golden jeweled crown, direct gaze, use of white and balanced mustache all are marks of the king in Balinese mask carving. Polychrome wood, hide, and hair, 7.25 inches.
Bali, Indonesia
Ca. mid 20th century
Collection of Jon and Cari Markell

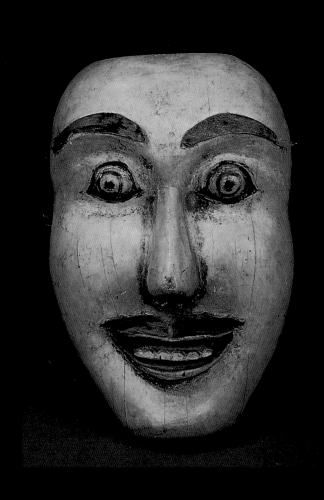 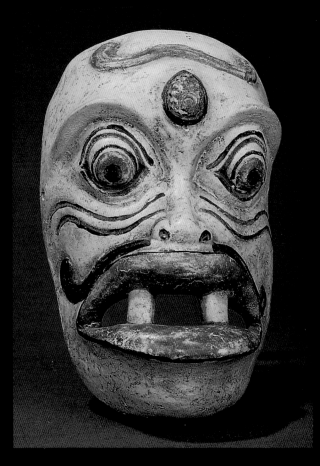 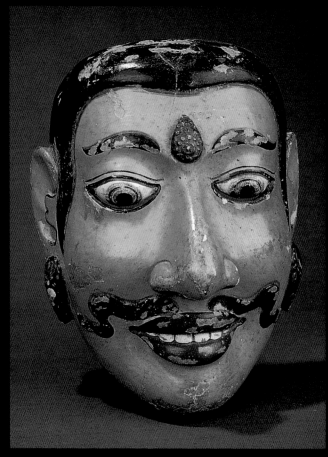

Topeng Telek
This is the mask of Sandara, one of the supporting players of the Barong (one of those on the good side.) Polychrome wood, animal hide, and hair, 7.25 inches.
Bali, Indonesia
Ca. mid 20th century
Collection of Jon and Cari Markell

Topeng Bonres
The Balinese also like to have fun and poke humor at themselves. This mask is of the clown-buffoon with an eccentric personality. Polychrome wood, 7 inches.
Bali, Indonesia
Ca. mid 20th century
Collection of Jon and Cari Markell

Face Mask
Mask used in Hindu-Animist Dance performance. Polychrome wood, 7.5 inches.
Bali, Indonesia
Ca. 19th century
Collection of Jerry Solomon, Los Angeles

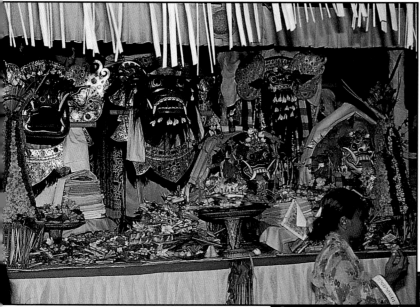

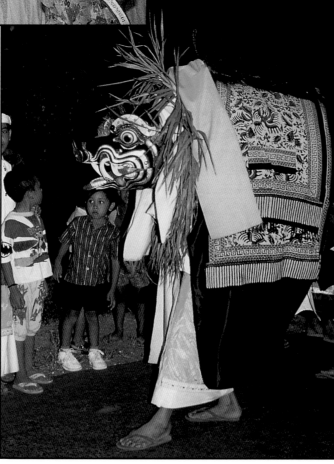

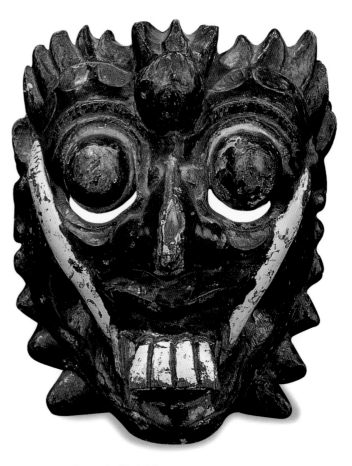

Above:
Altar Covered with Barong Masks.
The Barong protects the villages
from evil.
Bali, Indonesia
1993
Photo: Jim Pieper

Right:
Barong in an Evening Procession
Bali, Indonesia
1993
Photo: Jim Pieper

Rangda (Kala) Mask
The widow-witch associated with
destructive power, sickness, death
and the evil influence of black magic.
Polychrome wood, 9 inches.
Bali, Indonesia
Ca. 2nd quarter 20th century
Collection of Jon and Cari Markell

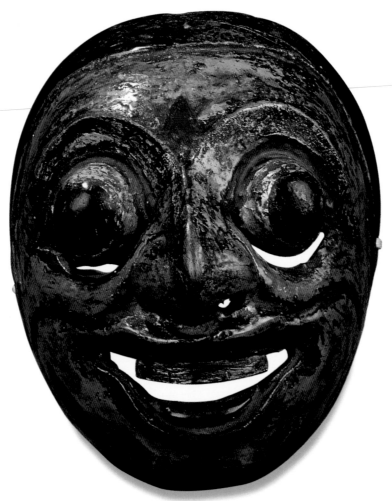

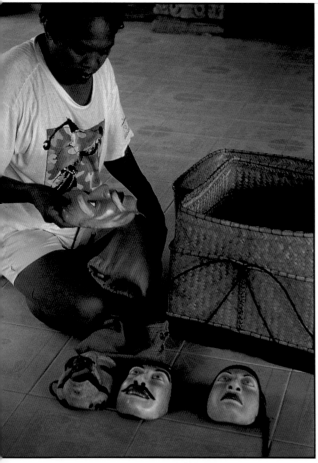

Balinese Dancer, Jimat Pedanda
One of Bali's leading dancers. At his grandfather's funeral, Pedanda danced as various traditional figures of Indonesian lore. Some of his dance masks are in the second generation of Pedanda's family and are carefully cared for, being stored in individual cloth bags between dances.
Bali, Indonesia
1993
Photo: Jim Pieper

Above:
Clown Mask
Oddball jokester who reveals the latest village gossip. Polychrome wood, 6.25 inches.
Bali or Lombok, Indonesia
Collection of Dr. John Ross

Right:
Laksmana Mask
Rama's younger brother who gives directions on morals and ethics. Polychrome wood, animal hide, hair, and mother-of-pearl, 7 inches.
Bali, Indonesia
Ca. 20th century
Collection of Dr. John Ross

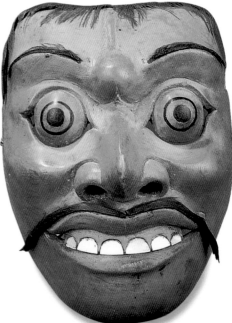

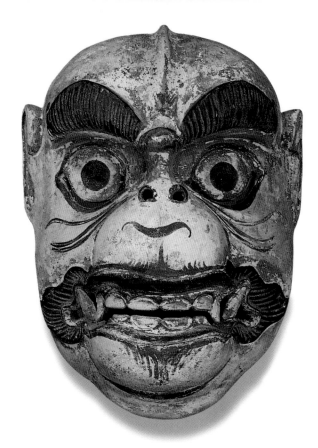

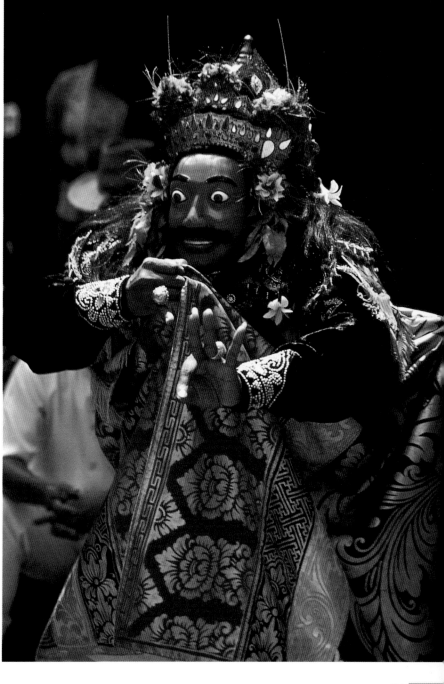

Left:
Topeng Subali
The white one, the wicked monkey brother of the monkey king in *Ramayana*. Polychrome wood, 8 inches.
Bali, Indonesia
Ca. mid 20th century
Collection of Jon and Cari Markell

Right:
Luh Semariani
Here Jimat Pedanda dancing as Luh Semariani
Bali, Indonesia
1993
Photo: Jim Pieper

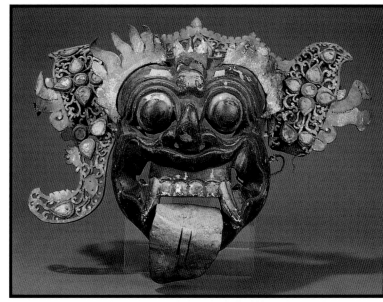

Rangda Mask
Polychrome wood, leather, metal, mirror, and paper, 10 inches.
Bali, Indonesia
Ca. late 19th to early 20th century
Collection of Dr. John Ross

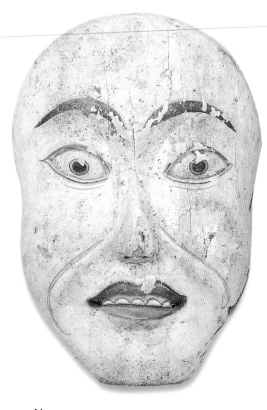

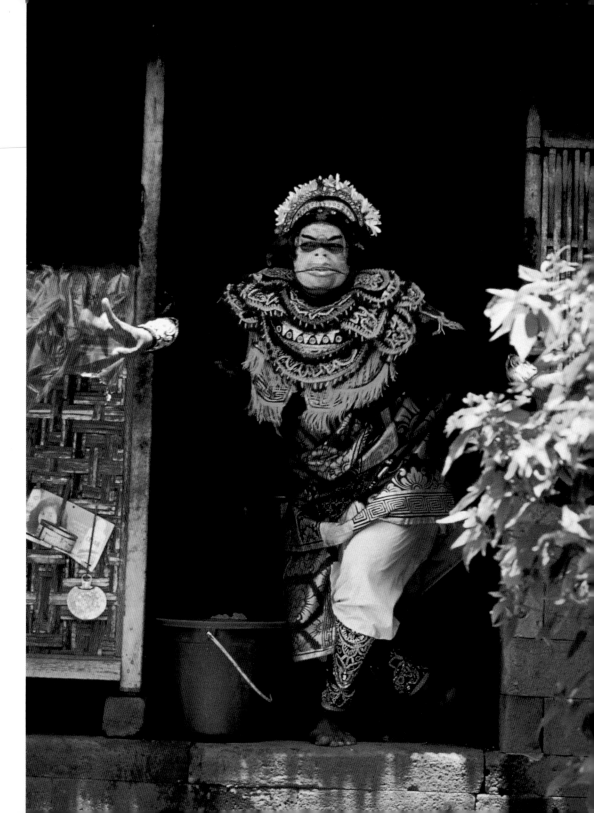

Above:
Dewi Sri
This small mask represents the goddess of rice, earth and fertility. The agricultural deity is believed to possess the power to make rice grow. It is placed on the bales of rice or in the home granary during festivals. Polychrome wood, 7 inches.
Bali, Indonesia
Ca. mid 20th century
Collection of Jon and Cari Markell

Right:
Sia Karya
Jimat Pedanda dancing as Sia Karya.
Bali, Indonesia
1993
Photo: Jim Pieper

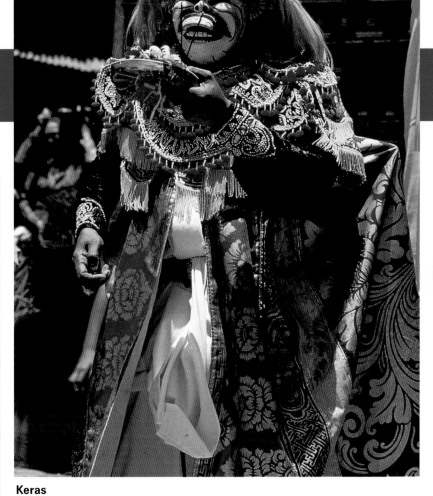

Keras
Pedanda dancing as Keras.
Bali, Indonesia
1993
Photo: Jim Pieper

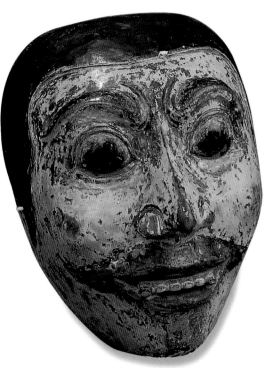

Telek Mask
Supporter of the Barong.
Polychrome wood, 7.75 inches.
Bali or Java, Indonesia
Collection of Dr. John Ross

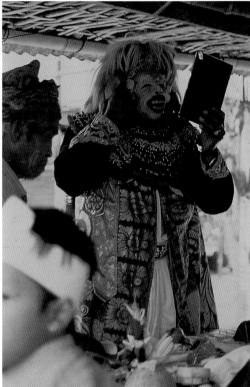

Pedanda checking his costume
before the dance.
Bali, Indonesia
1993
Photo: Jim Pieper

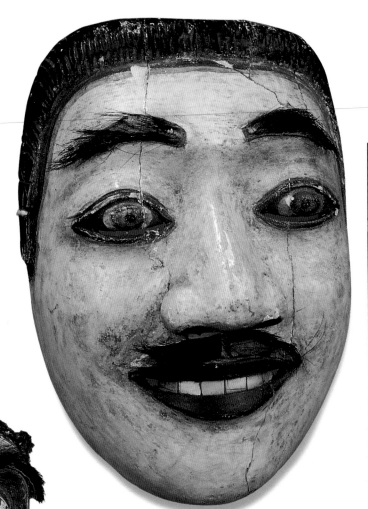

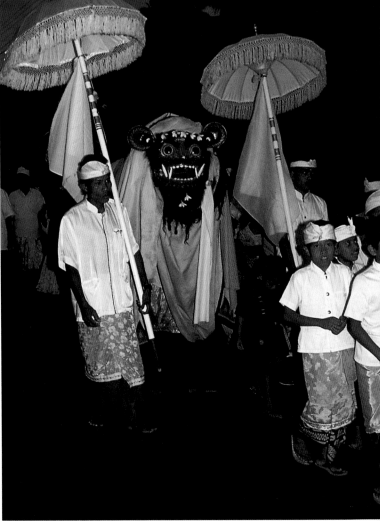

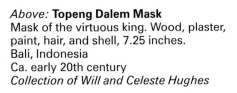

Above: **Topeng Dalem Mask**
Mask of the virtuous king. Wood, plaster,
paint, hair, and shell, 7.25 inches.
Bali, Indonesia
Ca. early 20th century
Collection of Will and Celeste Hughes

Left:
Deformity mask
Polychrome wood, skin with hair, and
shell, 7 inches.
Bali, Indonesia
Ca. mid 20th century
Collection of Dr. John Ross

Procession
Bali, Indonesia
1990s
Photo: Jim Pieper

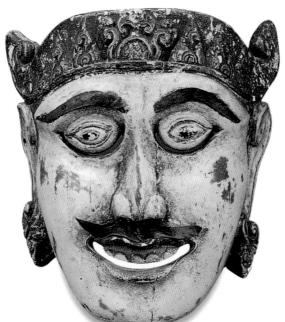

Topeng Dalem
The mask of the noble king, the white color denoting purity. Polychrome wood, and animal skin with hair, 7.75 inches.
Lombok, Indonesia
Ca. mid 20th century
Collection of Jon and Cari Markell

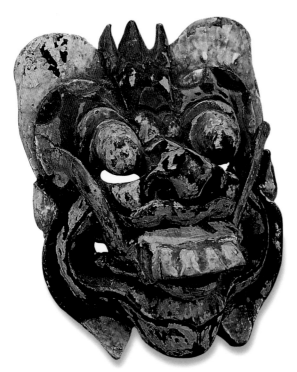

Topeng Rangda
This is a child's mask so they may learn about the widow-witch Rangda, the personification of all evil. Polychrome wood, 6.5 inches.
Lombok, Indonesia
Ca. mid 20th century
Collection of Jon and Cari Markell

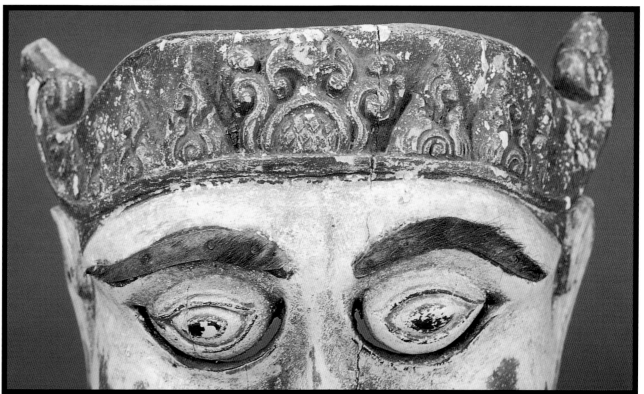

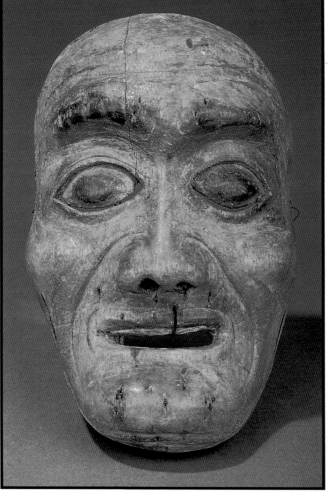

Topeng Tua (Old Man)
Extremely popular solo mask.
Polychrome wood, 8.75 inches.
Lombok, Indonesia
Ca. 20th century
Collection of Dr. John Ross

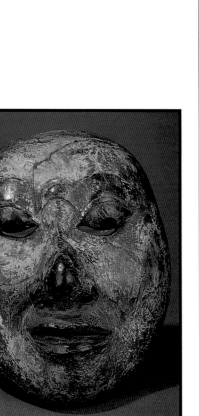

Dance Mask
Polychrome wood, 6.5 inches.
Lombok, Indonesia
Ca. 19th century
*Collection of Jerry Solomon,
Los Angeles*

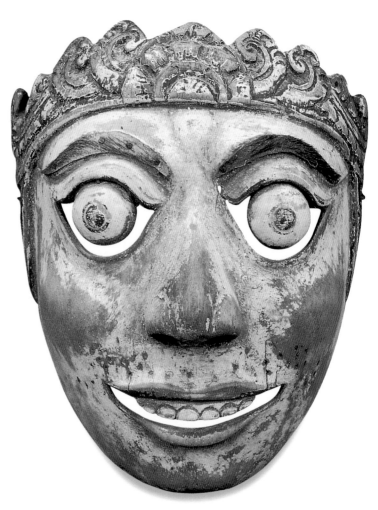

Topeng Dalem: The Virtuous King
Topeng is the dance drama of the Balinese
community in Lombok. Topeng literally means
"pressed against the face." Polychrome wood
and animal skin with hair, 7.25 inches.
Lombok, Indonesia
Ca. mid 20th century
Collection of Jon and Cari Markell

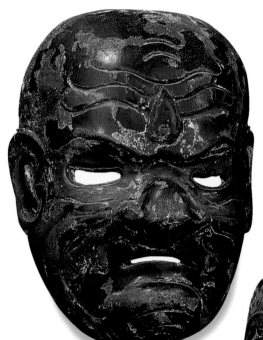

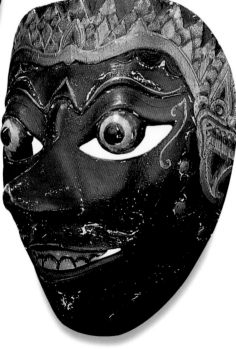

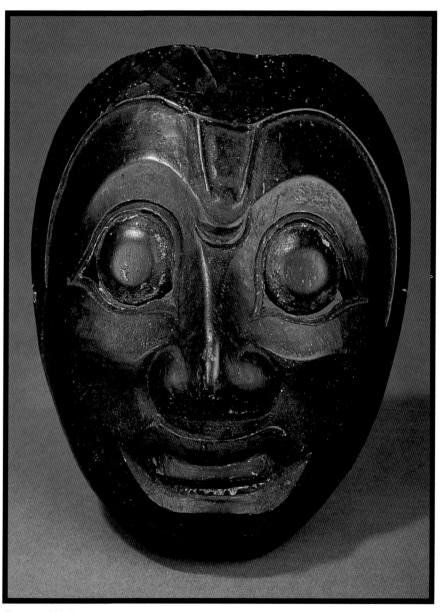

Above:
Topeng Tua
Old man influenced by the traditions of western neighbor Bali. Polychrome wood, 7.75 inches.
Lombok, Indonesia
Ca. early to mid 20th century
Collection of Jon and Cari Markell

Right:
Wayang Style Dance Mask
Polychrome wood, 7.25 inches.
Java, Indonesia
Ca. 1st quarter 20th century
Collection of Will and Celeste Hughes

Topeng Mask
Possibly in the form of Wayang. Polychrome wood, 7.25 inches.
Lombok or Java, Indonesia
Ca. 19th century
Collection of Jerry Solomon, Los Angeles

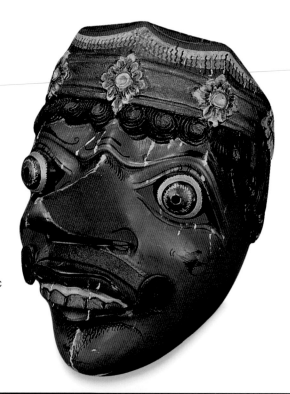

Demonic Character Mask
The grimace, large nose, and bulging eyes indicate that the mask represents a demonic character. The iconography is similar in Javanese shadow plays. Polychrome wood and leather, 7.25 inches.
Java, Indonesia
Ca. First Half 20th century
Collection Ann and Monroe Morgan

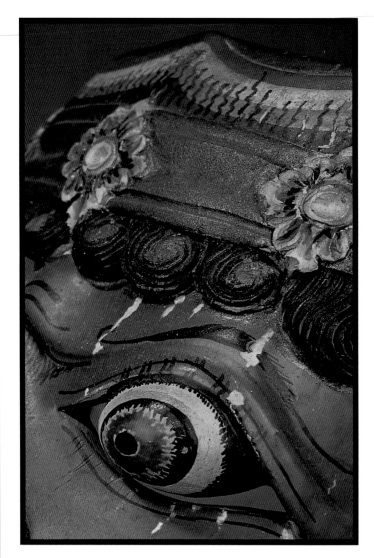

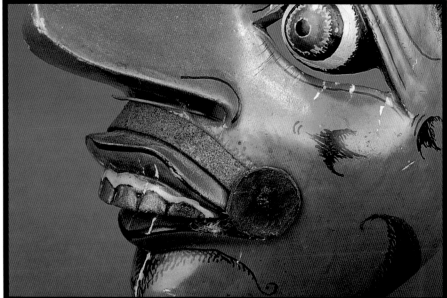

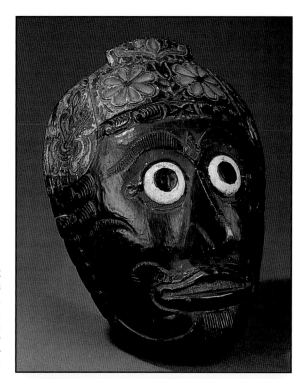

Wayan Topeng Mask
The character's name is
Bima. Polychrome wood,
8 inches.
Madura, Java, Indonesia
Ca. 19th century
*Collection of Jerry
Solomon, Los Angeles*

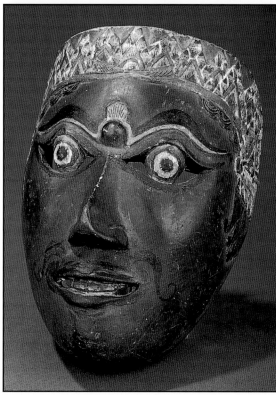

**Wayang-topeng Dance
Mask**
Polychrome wood,
7.75 inches.
Java, Indonesia
Ca. 1st quarter 20th century
*Collection of Will and
Celeste Hughes*

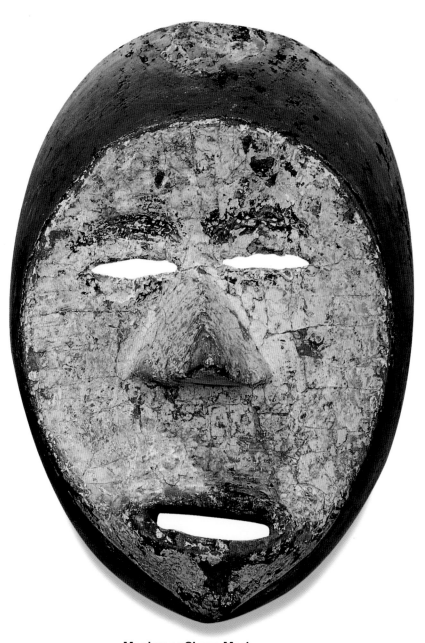

Monkey or Clown Mask
Polychrome wood, 7 inches.
Dieng Plateau Region, Central
Java, Indonesia
Ca. late 18th to early 19th century
Private Collection

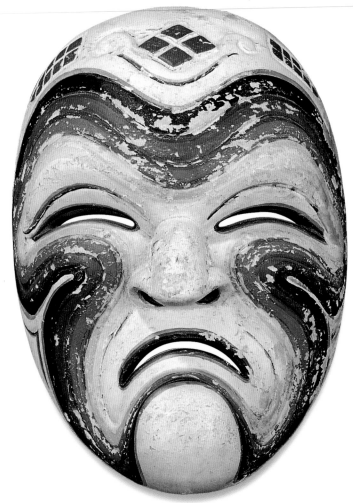

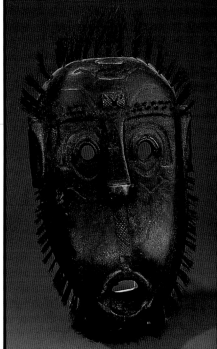

Monkey Mask
Wood and animal bristles,
13.5 inches.
Possibly Timor Island
Collection of Dr. John Ross

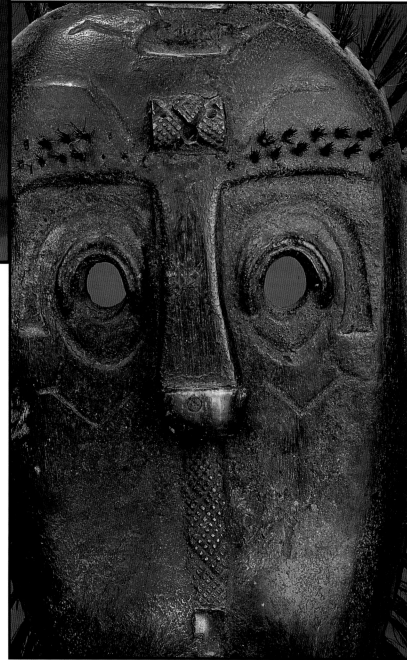

Topeng Tua
Old man copied after mask in the
Sultan of Yogjakarta's Palace.
Polychrome wood, 7 inches.
Java, Indonesia
Ca. early to mid 20th century
Collection of Jon and Cari Markell

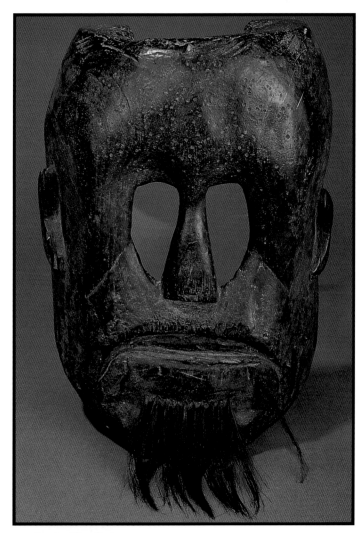

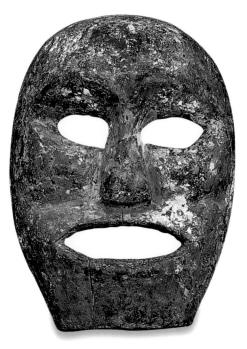

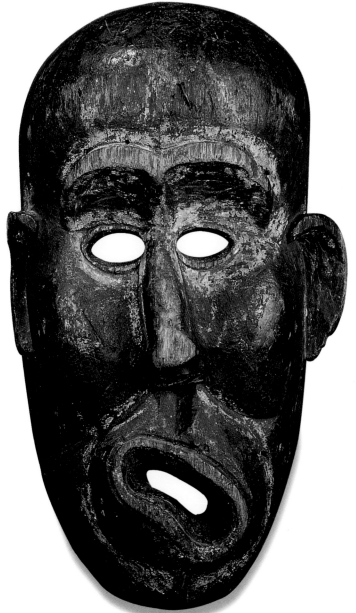

Above:
Ancestor Mask
The carving of ancestor masks is to placate potentially wrathful ancestral ghosts, who also have the power to grant fertility to men and woman.
Polychrome wood, 12.5 inches.
Atoni, West Timor, Indonesia
Ca. 3rd quarter 20th century
Collection of Jon and Cari Markell

Right:
Topong Mask
Polychrome wood, 14.25 inches.
Sumatra, Indonesia
Collection of Dr. John Ross

Beoto Marahuk
Ancestor Mask. Wood and hair, 11 inches.
Atoni, West Timor, Indonesia
Ca. 3rd quarter 20th century
Collection of Jon and Cari Markell

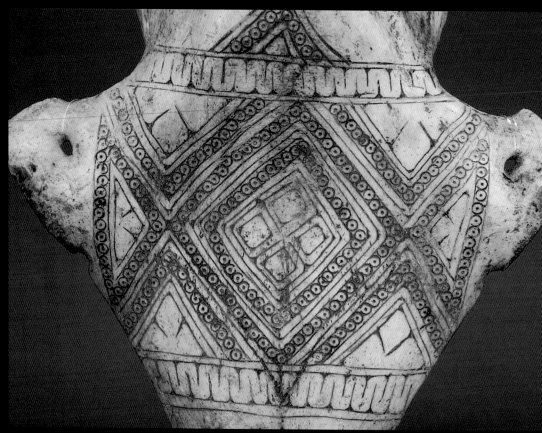

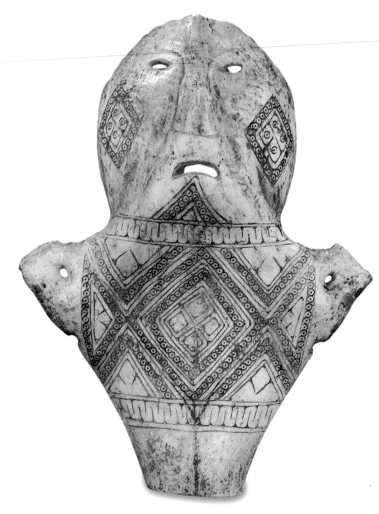

Skull Mask
Horse bone masks scare off evil spirits
while enhancing the spiritual and healing
powers of the shaman. Scrimshawed
bone, 8.75 inches.
Sumbanese People
Sumba, Indonesia
Ca. mid 20th century
Collection of Jim and Jeanne Pieper

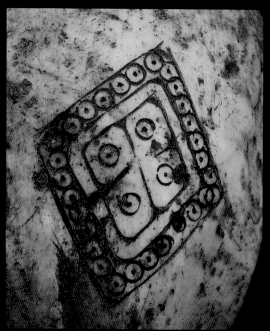

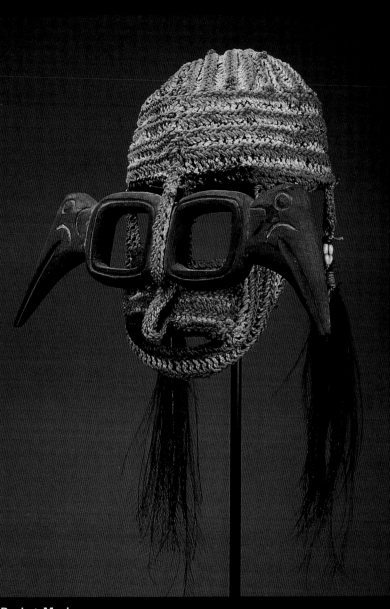

Basket Mask
Worn at the "Jipae" Festival. Woven fiber,
wood, feathers, twine, and shells, 11 inches.
Asmat People
Irian Jaya, Western New Guinea
Ca. late 20th century
Collection of Shirley and David Rowen

PHILIPPINES

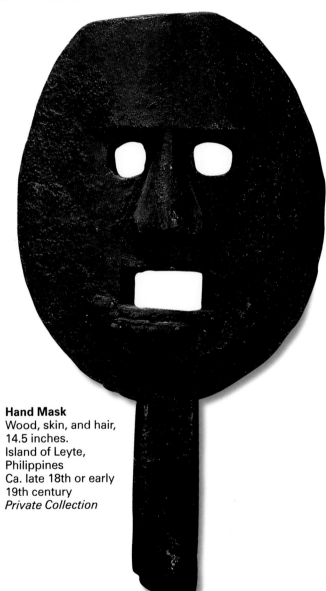

Hand Mask
Wood, skin, and hair,
14.5 inches.
Island of Leyte,
Philippines
Ca. late 18th or early
19th century
Private Collection

105

MELANESIA: PAPUA NEW GUINEA

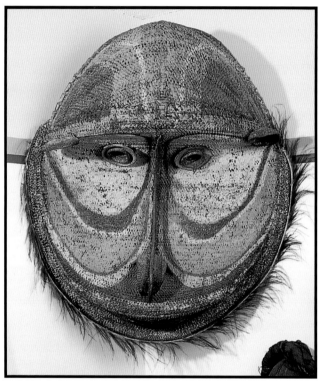

Gable Mask
This mask was hung on the gable of the men's meeting house, under the eaves. It provided protection from evil spirits for the male elders during their meetings. Basketry, paint, and feathers, 38 inches.
Maprik People
Sepik River, New Guinea
Ca. 2nd quarter 20th century
Collection of Diane and Ernie Wolfe III

Below:
Yam Mask
Woven fiber, paint, 11.75 inches.
Ca. 1970
Abelam People

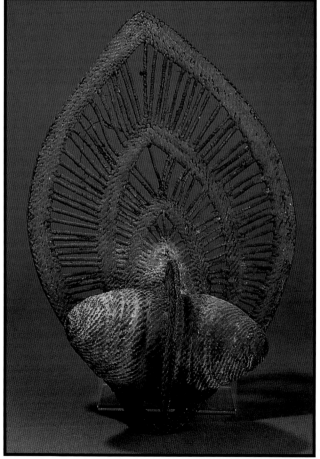

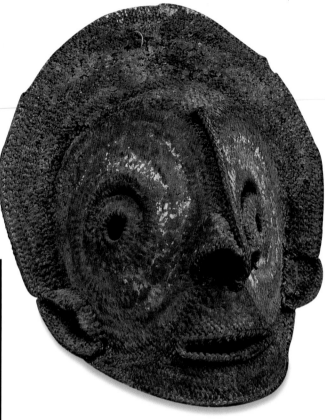

Above:
Yam Mask
Masks are used to cover long yams in a ceremony showing the men's gardening prowess. It is of utmost importance in the culture. The Abelam believe only men can grow long yams. Their success is dependent not only on hard work, but complete abstinance from contact with women during the sixth month growing period, and spiritual assistance from ancestors. A fine yam is named for the ancestral spirit and that spirit is brought into being by the mask and decoration. Woven fiber, paint, 9.75 inches.
Ca. 1960
Abelam People
Southern Abelam Area, Papua New Guinea
Collection of Michael Hamson

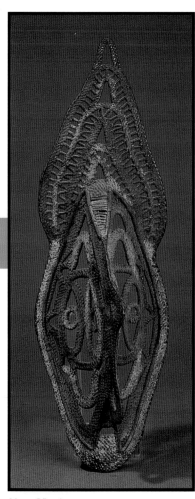

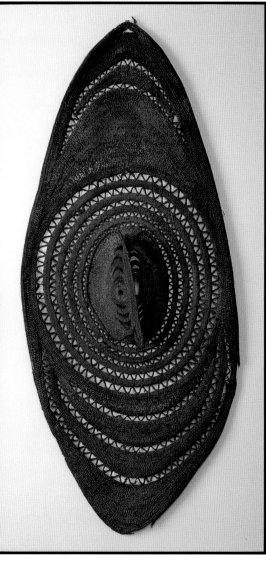

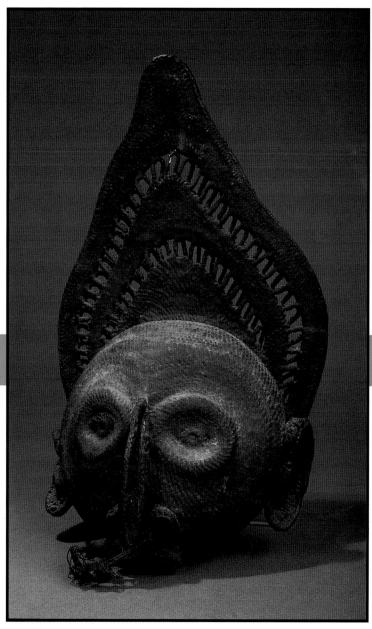

Yam Mask
Woven fiber, 36 inches.
Ca. 1970
Abelam People
Southern Abelam Area, Papua New Guinea
Collection of Michael Hamson

Yam Mask
Woven fiber, paint, 14.75 inches.
Ca. 1960
Abelam People
Southern Abelam Area, Papua
New Guinea
Collection of Michael Hamson

Yam Mask
Woven fiber, and paint, 13.5 inches.
Ca. 1960
Abelam People
Southern Abelam Area, Papua New Guinea
Collection of Michael Hamson

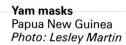

Yam masks
Papua New Guinea
Photo: Lesley Martin

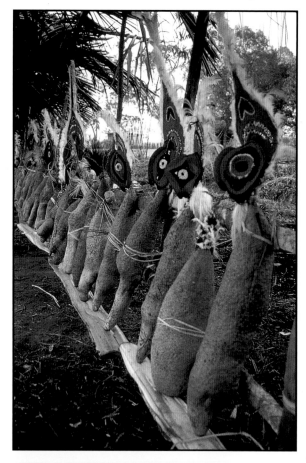

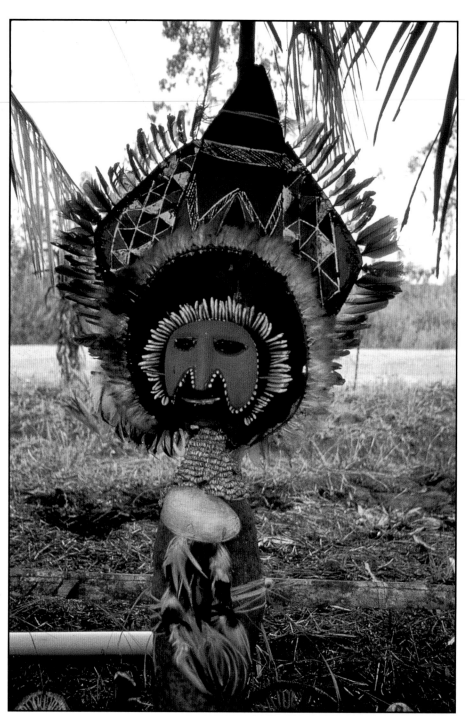

I collect ethnographic art because it expresses the vast diversity of human experience at the same time as reminding me of the basic humanity shared by all cultures.
Michael Hamson

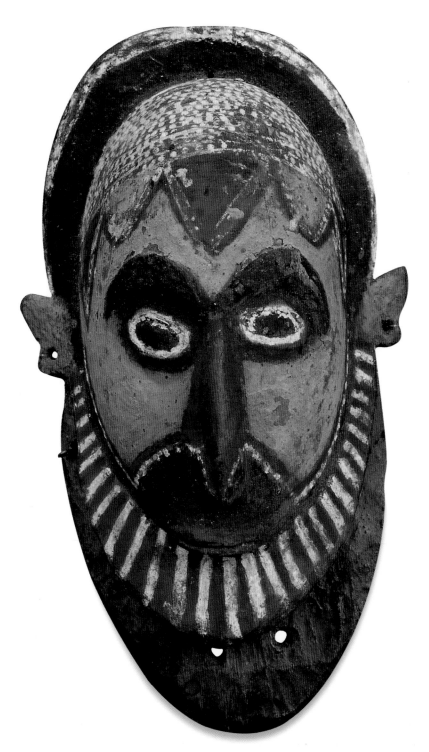

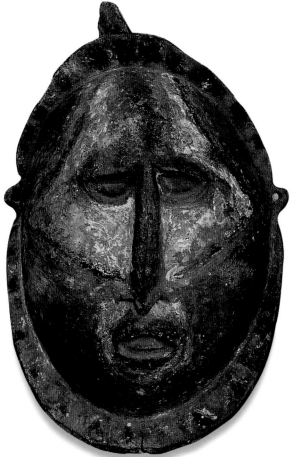

Above:
Yam Mask
Polychrome wood, 10.5 inches.
Ca. 1925
Abelam People
Southern Abelam Area, Papua New Guinea
Collection of Michael Hamson

Left:
Yam Mask
Some hardwood masks are also used to
decorate the ceremonial yams. Wood is used
more frequently in Southern and Eastern
Abelam. Polychrome wood, 8.5 inches.
Ca. 1980
Yamis Village, East Sepik, Papua, New Guinea
Collection of Michael Hamson

*Collecting is moments
of time that can extend to
days of excitement to ac-
quire, accumulate, own
and, yes, display. It is the
finding of a treasure per-
ceived to be of value only
by yourself, and the won-
der of being trusted with
the history and the es-
sence of others. It is to
have the opportunity to
know, feel and sense the
spirituality of humankind's
creative hand.*
Jeanne and Jim Pieper

Parak (Mosquito Nose) Mask
This particular mask has a personal name of "Windigawa." Masks were used in both male initiation ceremonies and rituals concerned with the growing of yams. Polychrome wood, 17.5 inches. Sereng Village, Boken Plains, Papua New Guinea Ca. 2nd quarter 20th century *Collection of Michael Hamson*

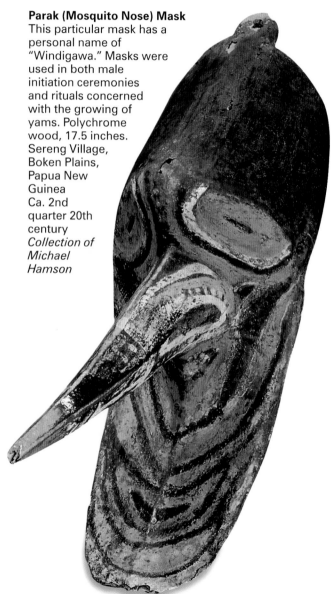

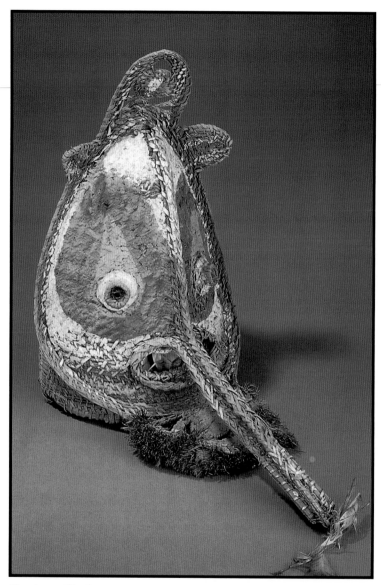

Tumbuan Mask
The elongated nose is a symbol of virility. This mask was used to scare women and children away from the site of male initiation ceremonies *(Maksic, PANG, p. 25)*. Woven fiber, natural fibers, feathers, twine, and paint, 21.5 inches. Sangriman, Papua, New Guinea Ca. mid 20th century *Collection of Mr. and Mrs. David E. Hayen*

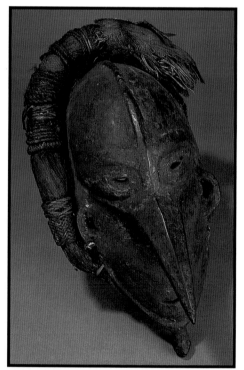

Lewa Masks
Masks were attached to conical headdresses and worn by men whose role it was to impose restrictions on certain foodstuffs in preparation for a communal feast. The spirit manifested by these masks was called "Tangbwal." Wood, natural fiber, twine, and woven fiber, 15.5 inches. Vokeo Island, Papua New Guinea Ca. 1st quarter 20th century *Collection of Michael Hamson*

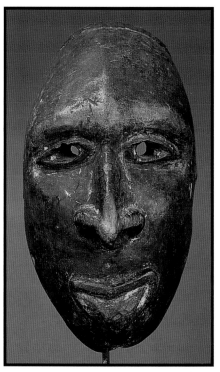

Canoe Bow Mask
Wood, 9 inches.
Coastal region, between Keram
and Ramu Rivers, New Guinea
Collection of Dr. John Ross

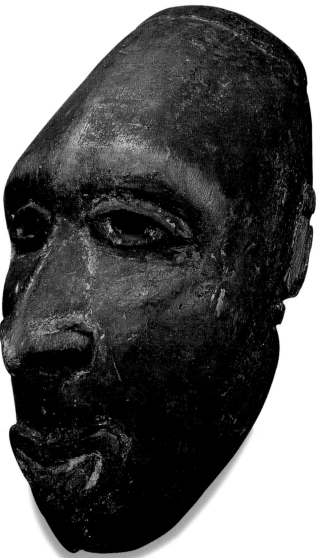

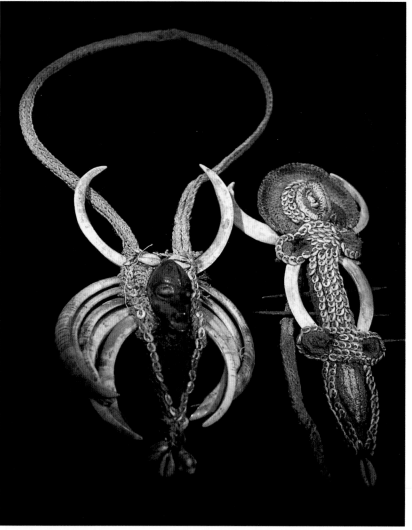

Karavt or Antikara
Protective amulets worn by men to please ancestral spirits.
Left: a very rare miniature Wood Spirit mask with bore tusks,
which also adorns men in battle. Boiken People, Hapmogun,
New Guinea. **Right:** a miniature yam mask which is also used to
adorn the yams during the annual ceremonies.
Abelan People.
Ca. mid 20th century
Collection of Jim and Jeanne Pieper.

ENGLAND

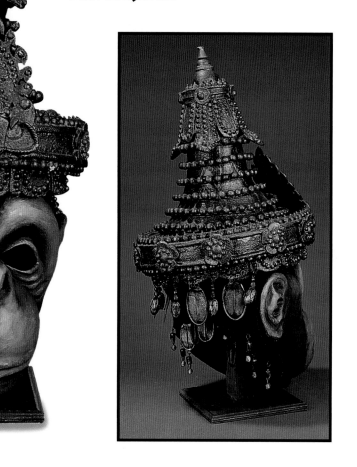

Hanuman Monkey King Mask
Hanuman is a god in the Indian epic, the *Ramayana.* He is the ally of Rama and is still worshipped in India. The mask was worn in the play "Mono-logues in Front of Burning Cities" at the Old Vic in London. The play is about Indian mutiny. Composite, cloth, and metal, 20.5 inches.
Made in India, used in theater in London, United Kingdom
Ca. 3rd quarter 20th century
Collection of Ann and Monroe Morgan

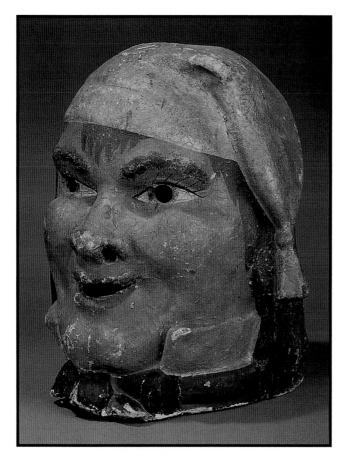

FRANCE

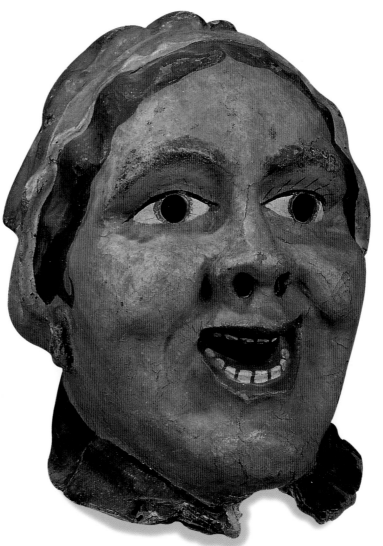

Above:
French Carnival Helmet
Peasant man. Polychrome composite,
12 inches.
France
Ca. early 20th century
Collection of Ann and Monroe Morgan

Right:
French Carnival Helmet
Peasant woman. Composite, 12 inches.
France
Ca. early 20th century
Collection of Ann and Monroe Morgan

AUSTRIA

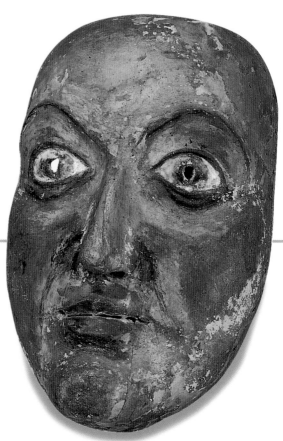

Devil Mask
In the Alpine region, masks fall into two categories: beautiful and ugly. The ugly are usually witches or devils. A devil like this one is based on the Christian idea of a devil, a la Durer. Often used in theatrical plays. Polychrome wood, 17.5 inches.
Tyrol, Austria
Ca. late 19th or early 20th century
Collection of Ann and Monroe Morgan

GERMANY

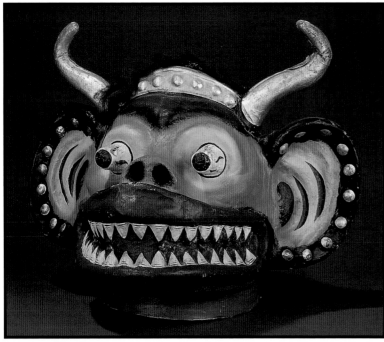

Carnival Mask
Grinning cow head monster. Papier mâché, cotton, fabric, and hair, 17 inches.
Germany
Ca. early 20th century
Collection of Ann and Monroe Morgan

SWITZERLAND

Carnival Mask
Alpine festivals are traditional with much merrymaking and mocking of authority. The characters are fools, witches (the ugly), or Hansels (the beautiful). Polychrome wood, 9 inches.
Switzerland
Ca. late 19th century
Collection of Ann and Monroe Morgan

ITALY

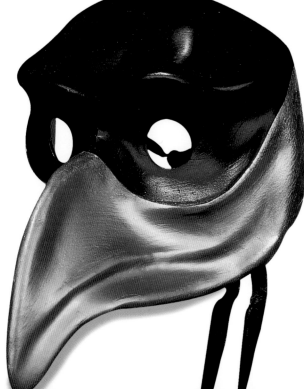

Dottore (Doctor) Mask
Made by Givliana Bortolodini
Dottore walks around at Carnival wearing a black gown and carrying a white stick like a baton. In medieval times, the stick was to lift the sheets of a patient so that Dottore would not get contaminated. Papier mâché, 15 inches.
Venice, Italy
Ca. late 20th century
Collection of Shirley and David Rowen

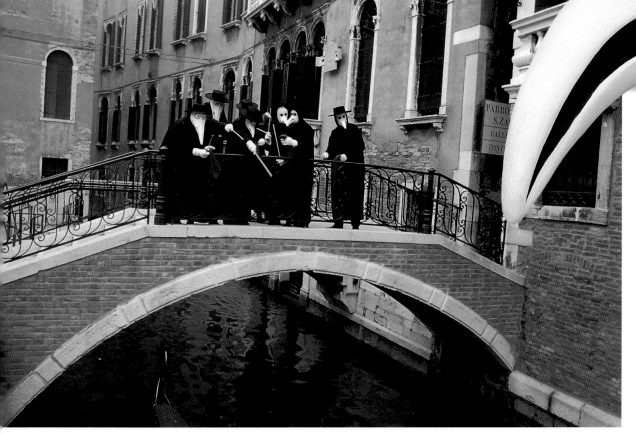

Dottore (Doctor) Mask
Venice, Italy
Photo: Shirley and David Rowen

Bird Carnival Mask
Papier mâché, 8.25 inches.
Venice, Italy
Ca. late 20th century
Collection of Shirley and David Rowen

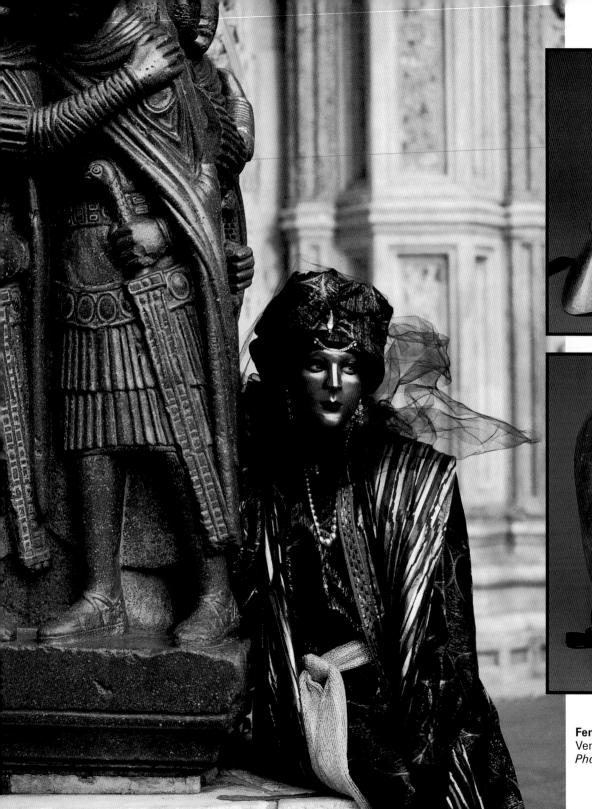

Carnival Mask
Gold traditional "Bituta" mask, worn by men and women. Most popular mask of the Venice carnival. Papier mâché and ribbon, 7.5 inches.
Venice, Italy
Ca. late 20th century
Collection of Shirley and David Rowen

Female Carnival Mask
Composite, 8.75 inches.
Venice, Italy
Ca. late 20th century
Collection of Shirley and David Rowen

Female Carnival Mask
Venice, Italy
Photo: Shirley and David Rowen

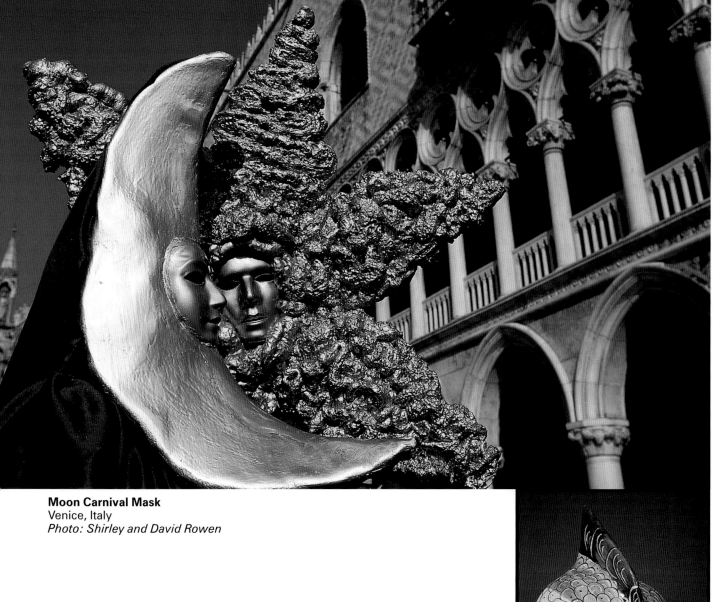

Moon Carnival Mask
Venice, Italy
Photo: Shirley and David Rowen

Parrot Carnival Mask
Papier mâché, 13.5 inches.
Venice, Italy
Ca. late 20th century
*Collection of Shirley and
David Rowen*

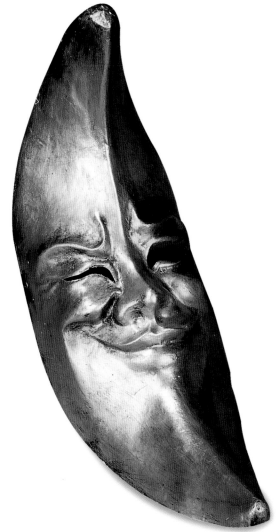

Moon Carnival Mask
Papier mâché and ribbon,
21.25 inches.
Venice, Italy
Ca. late 20th century
*Collection of Shirley and
David Rowen*

117

THE AMERICAS

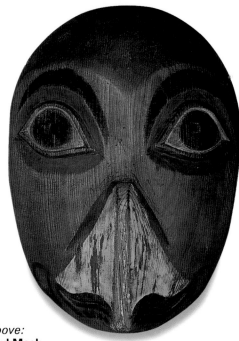

CANADA

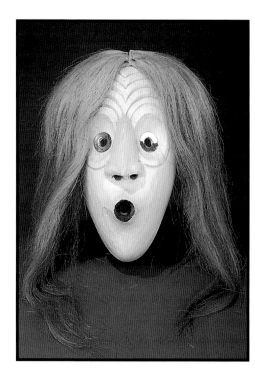

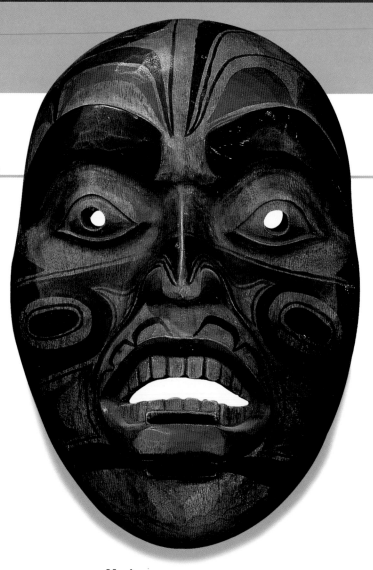

Above:
Bird Mask
Possibly an eagle. Polychrome wood, 9 inches.
Haida People
British Colombia, Canada
Ca. late 19th century
Collection of Joni and Monte Gordon,
Newspace, Los Angeles

Right:
Whistler Mask
Carved by Dehandra. Polychrome wood, animal hair, and metal, 12 inches.
Wolf Clan
Cayuga, Iroquois Six Nations
Canada
Ca. mid 20th century
Collection of Annette and Seymour Bird

Mask
Polychrome wood, 11.5 inches.
Kwakiutl People
British Columbia, Canada
Ca. mid 20th century
Collection of Joni and Monte Gordon,
Newspace, Los Angeles

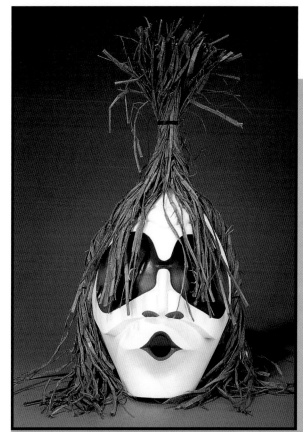

Festival Mask
Carved by Alexander Joseph. Polychrome wood, and cedar shavings, 21 inches.
Salisi People
Canada
Ca. late 20th century
Collection of Annette and Seymour Bird

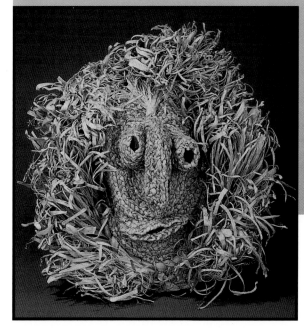

Corn Husk Mask
The Husk Faces were farmers who lived on the other side of the earth. Each year they visited the Seneca Long House during two nights of mid-winter festival. They were messengers of three sisters: Corn, Squash and Beans. They also had curing powers. Corn husk, 12 inches.
Canada
Ca. 1974
Collection Ann and Monroe Morgan

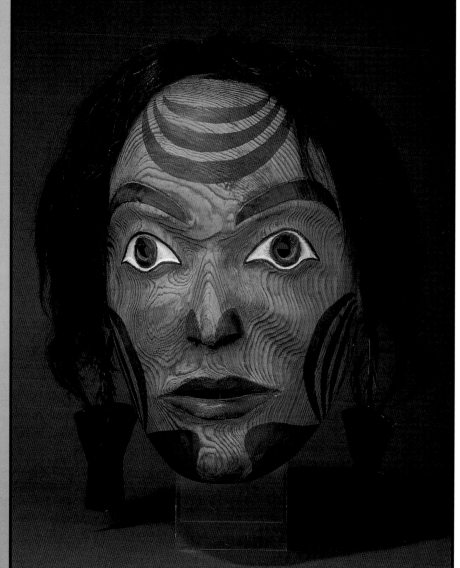

Portrait Mask
In Haida the word for mask means to imitate. Some masks are abstractions, and some, like this one are very realistic portrayals of real people, usually ancestors. *(TSW, p. 104)* Polychrome wood and hair, 10.75 inches.
Haida People
British Columbia, Canada
Ca. mid 20th century
Collection of Annette and Seymour Bird

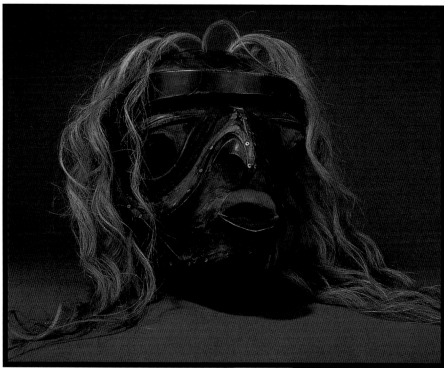

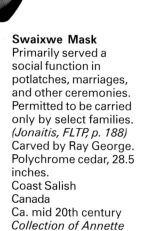

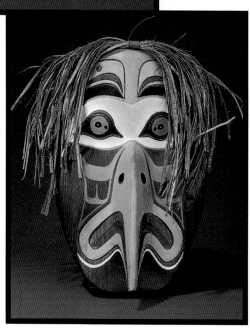

Above:
Hawk Mask
The guardian spirit of the chief.
(Bruggmann, p. 116, pl. 71) Polychrome
wood and hair, 8.5 inches.
Kwakiutl People
Northwest Coast, Canada
Ca. late 19th to early 20th century
Collection of Joni and Monte Gordon,
Newspace, Los Angeles

Right:
Eagle Mask
Polychrome cedar and cedar shavings,
14.5 inches.
Northwest Coast People
Canada
Ca. late 20th century
Collection of Dr. Harry and Claire
Steinberg

Swaixwe Mask
Primarily served a
social function in
potlatches, marriages,
and other ceremonies.
Permitted to be carried
only by select families.
(Jonaitis, FLTP, p. 188)
Carved by Ray George.
Polychrome cedar, 28.5
inches.
Coast Salish
Canada
Ca. mid 20th century
Collection of Annette
and Seymour Bird

THE UNITED STATES

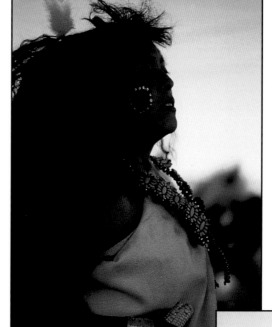

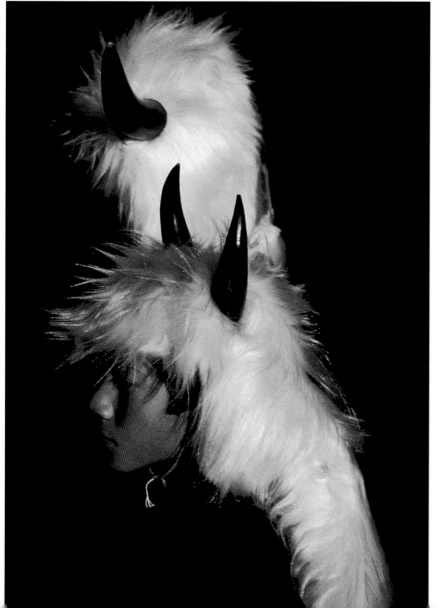

Zuni Dancers in the White Buffalo Dance
The girl does not wear a mask in the White Buffalo dance, but face paint only. The dance is considered a social dance and may be photographed.
1990s
Photos: Jim Pieper

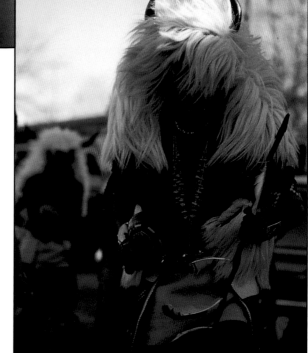

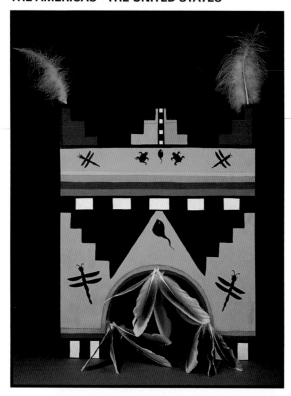

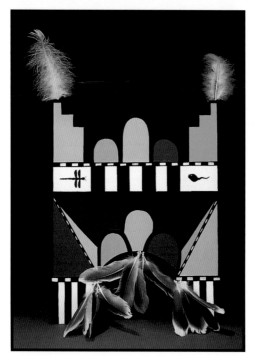

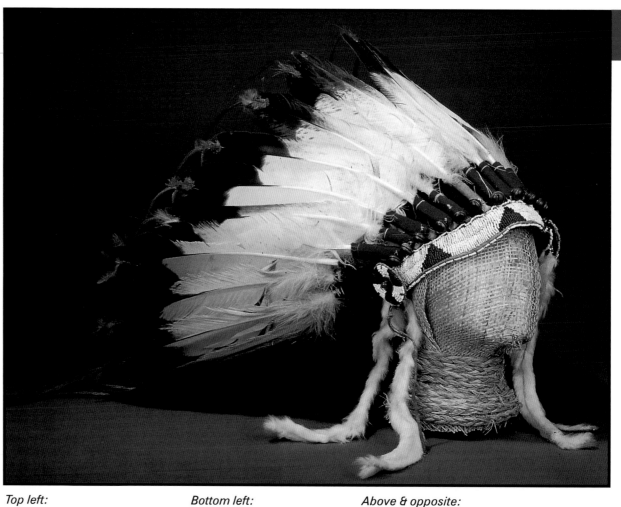

Top left:
Tableta
Polychrome wood and feathers, 17.75 inches.
Zuni People
New Mexico, United States
Ca. 1990
Collection of Jim and Jeanne Pieper
Gifted to Amerind Foundation, Inc.

Bottom left:
Tableta
Polychrome wood and feathers, 17.5 inches.
Zuni People
New Mexico, United States
Ca. 1990
Collection of Jim and Jeanne Pieper
Gifted to Amerind Foundation, Inc.

Above & opposite:
Sioux Head Dress and Shirt
This ceremonial costume was owned by the lender's Sioux father. The headdress is constructed of eagle and other feathers, wool, bells, beads, leather, and rabbit skin, 16 inches high at the front. The shirt is made of leather, beads, human hair, 35 inches long and 18 inches wide at the shoulders.
Sioux People
Rosebud, South Dakota, United States
Ca. early 20th century
Collection of Kent Valandra

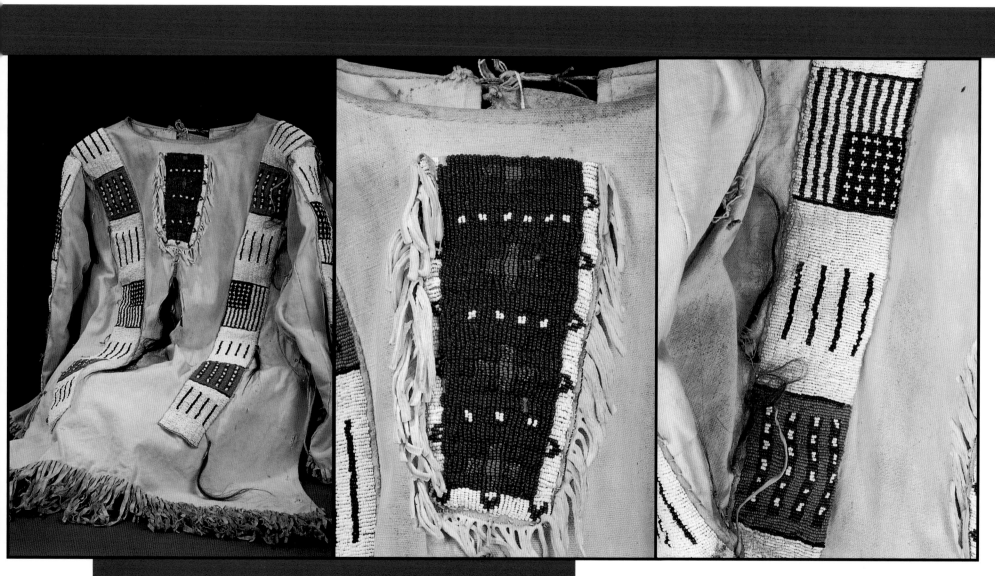

We have always been drawn to and enriched by folk art. It is both exciting to buy and to explore the meanings and traditions behind it. When we look at our collection, we see we are surrounded by faces, in the figures and the puppets, and of course the masks. Each one has a story, a drama and a magic.
Ann and Monroe Morgan

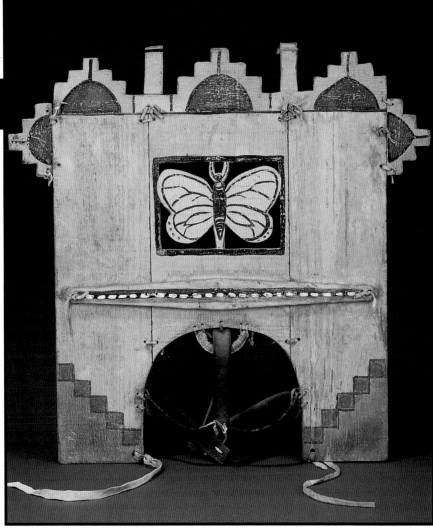

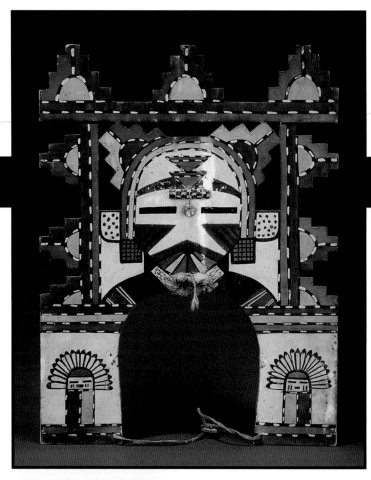

Palhik Mana Butterfly Tableta
Polychrome wood and plant fibers, 17 inches.
Hopi People
Arizona, United States
Ca. 1970
Collection of Jim and Jeanne Pieper Gifted to Amerind Foundation, Inc.

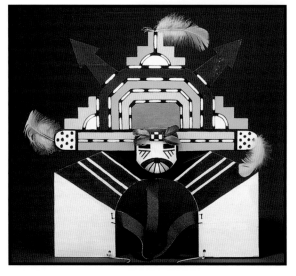

Poli Mana or ButterflyTableta
Hopi Butterfly tableta. Polychrome wood, cord, and leather, 20 inches.
Hopi People
Arizona, United States
Ca. mid 20th century
Collection of Jim and Jeanne Pieper

Kopachuki Child's Tableta
Polychrome wood, feathers, and leather, 16 inches.
Hopi People
3rd Mesa, Arizona, United States
Ca. 1995
Collection of Jim and Jeanne Pieper

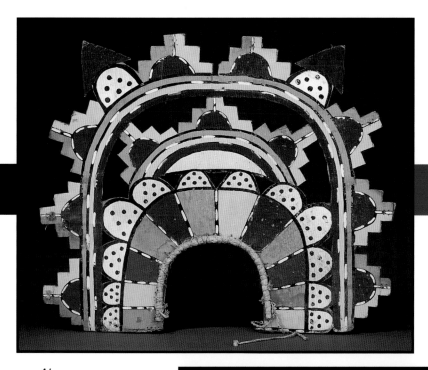

Note: The Hopi masks shown on this and following pages were part of a collection that was destroyed in a fire. Only the photographs remain.

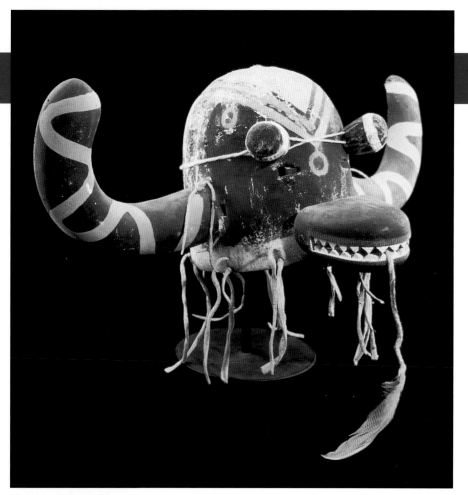

Above:
Butterfly Tableta
Polychrome on corru-
gated board with fibers
and string, 19.5 inches.
Hopi People
Arizona, United States
Ca. 1950
*Collection of Jim and
Jeanne Pieper
Gifted to Amerind
Foundation, Inc.*

Right:
**Navan or Velvet Shirt
Helmet Mask**
Also known as the
Navan Kachina, it
appears in regular
Kachina dances. Also
part of the Zuni
pantheon. *(Colton 171,
p. 60)*
Hopi People
Hopi, Arizona, U.S.
Ca. mid 20th century
*Private collection
Photo: Jim Pieper*

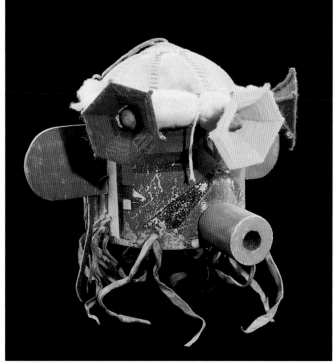

Ho-o-te Helmet Mask
Appears in Mixed Kachina Dance, carrying bow and
arrows, and rattle. The dancer's body is painted red with
yellow shoulders, forearms, and lower legs. *(Colton
104, p. 44)* Believed to be able to forecast spring.
Hopi People
Hopi, Arizona, United States
Ca. mid 20th century.
*Private collection
Photo: Jim Pieper*

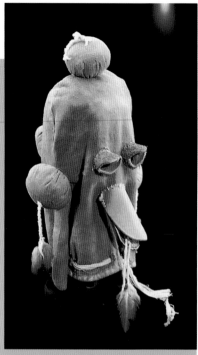

Left:
Koyemsi or Mudhead Helmet Mask
Koyemsi or the Mudhead Clown is the sometimes referred to as a Hopi Clown. The body and mask are covered in red clay. *(Colton 59, p. 34)*
Hopi People
Possibly First Mesa Hopi, Arizonia, U.S.
Private collection
Photo: Jim Pieper

Below:
Ahul or Ahola Helmet Mask
The Chief Kachina, Ahul is the Solstice or Return Kachina. Appears in agricultural dances to insure strong crops. *(Wright, p. 36, Colton 2, p. 20)*
The Hopi People
Hopi, Arizona, United States
Ca. 19th century
Private collection
Photo: Jim Pieper

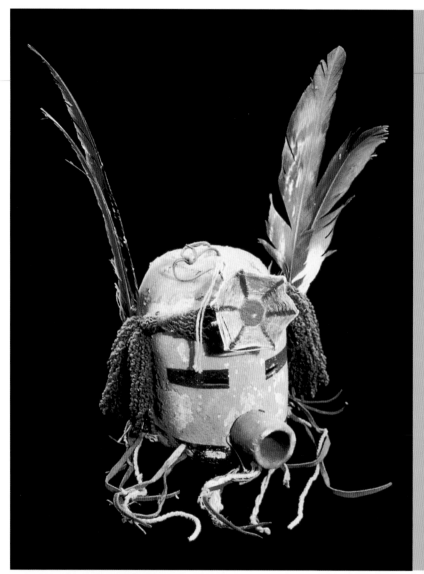

Kahaila or Kwasus Alek Taka
Hunter Helmet Mask *(Colton 145, p. 54).*
Hopi People
Hopi, Arizona, United States
Ca. mid 20th century
Private collection
Photo: Jim Pieper

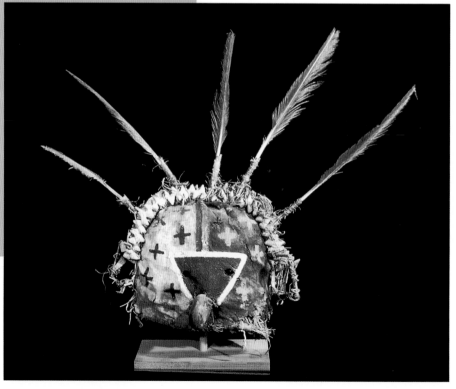

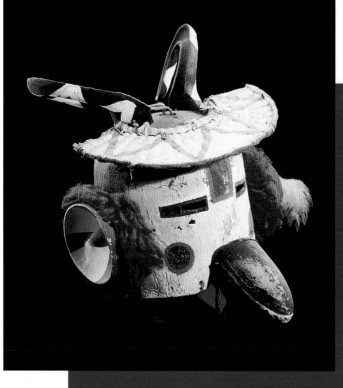

"Chof" Antelope Helmet Mask
Believed to have the power to bring rain, vegetation, and the game that follows. May also have curative powers. *(Colton 90, p. 41)*
Hopi People
Hopi, Arizona, United States
Ca. mid 20th century
Private collection
Photo: Jim Pieper

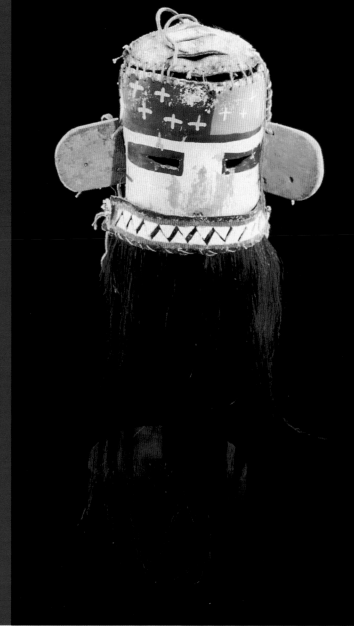

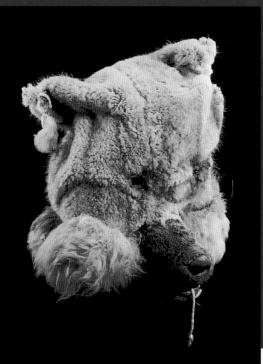

"Kweo" Wolf Helmet Mask
Helmet made of carpet utilizing a much older cottonwood carved nose and mouth. *(Colton 86, p. 40)*
Hopi People
Hopi, Arizona
Ca. mid 20th century
Private collection
Photo: Jim Pieper

Possibly Hititi Helmet Mask
Protector against witchcraft.
Hopi People
Hopi, Arizona, United States
Ca. early 20th century
Private collection
Photo: Jim Pieper

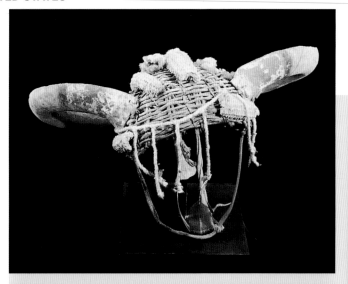

Two Horned Priest's Hat
Made of very old woven
cap with corn cobs,
cotton, and cut gourd
horns, and painted with
natural mineral paints.
Hopi People
First Mesa, Hopi, Arizona,
United States
Ca. 19th century
Private collection
Photo: Jim Pieper

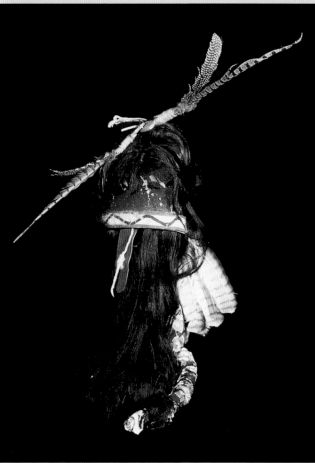
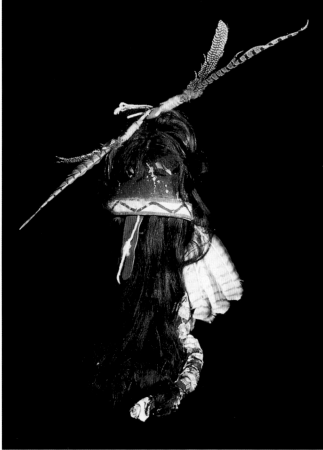

"Chakwaina" Face Mask
Taken from the Zuni and
brought to First Mesa,
Chakwaina is a warrior
kachina, found in many
pueblos. *(Wright, p. 34;*
Colton 160 p. 57)
Hopi People
Hopi, Arizona, United
States
Ca. mid 20th century
Private collection
Photo: Jim Pieper

"Susopa" Cricket Helmet Mask
(Colton 64, p. 35)
Hopi People
Hopi, Arizona, United States
Ca. mid 20th century
Private collection
Photo: Jim Pieper

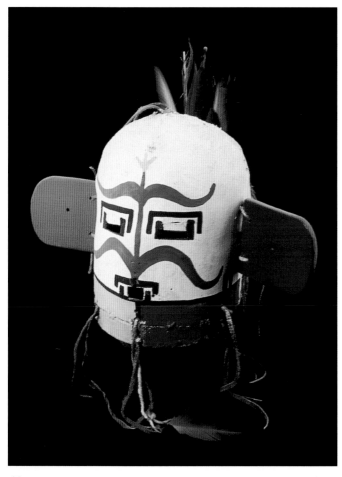

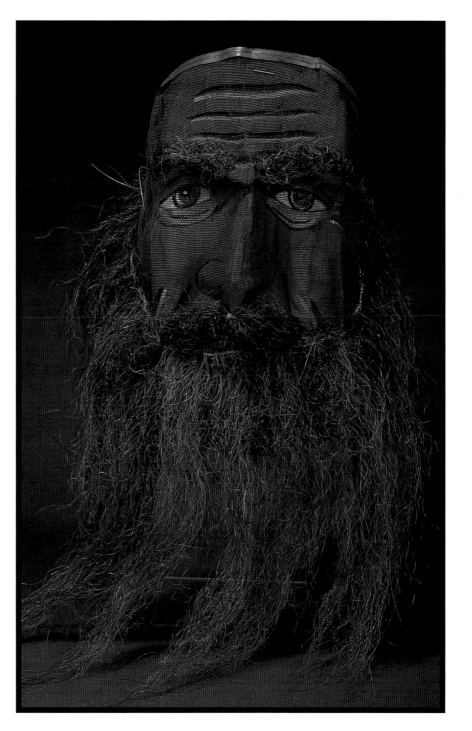

Above:
Tasaf Yebitchai or Navajo Talking God Helmet Mask
This kachina was taken from the Navajo culture. *(Colton 139, p. 52)*
Hopi People
First Mesa, Hopi, Arizona, United States
Ca. mid 20th century
Private collection
Photo: Jim Pieper

Right:
Odd Fellows Lodge Mask
The Order of Odd Fellows is a secret benevolent society with mystic signs of recognition, initiation rites, and ceremonies.
Metallic mesh and fiber, 13.5 inches overall.
Ca. early 20th century
Seattle, Washington
Collection Ann and Monroe Morgan

Left to right:

Animal and Bird Masks
Mardi Gras cloth masks designed by Gayle Stancil, shown holding the bird mask.
Maskmaker: Lafayette, Louisiana
Mardi Gras: New Orleans, Louisiana
1999
Photo: Jim Pieper

Bird Mask
Mardi Gras
Designed by Gayle Stancil
New Orleans, Louisiana
1999
Photo: Jim Pieper

Feather Mask
Mardi Gras
New Orleans, Louisiana
1999
Photo: Jim Pieper

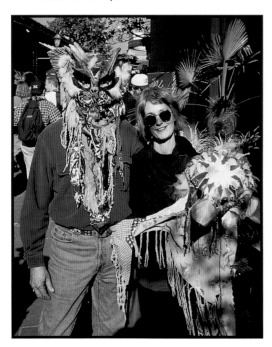

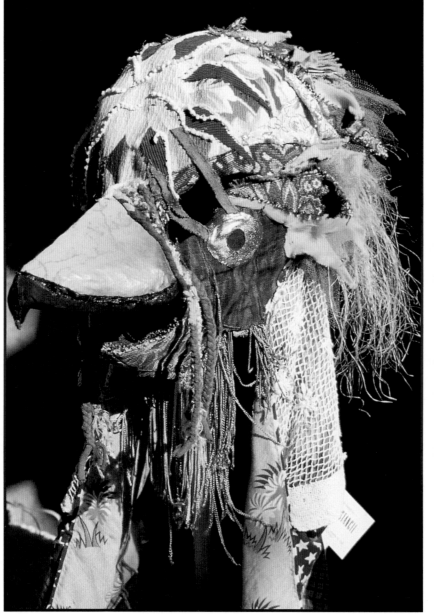

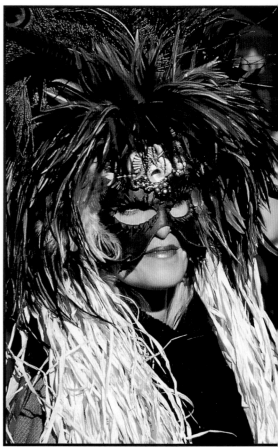

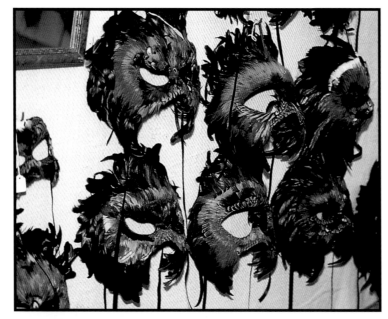

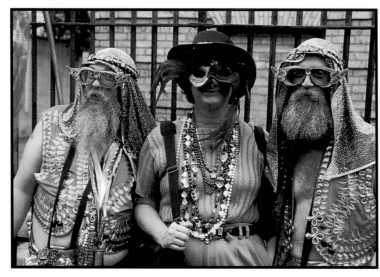

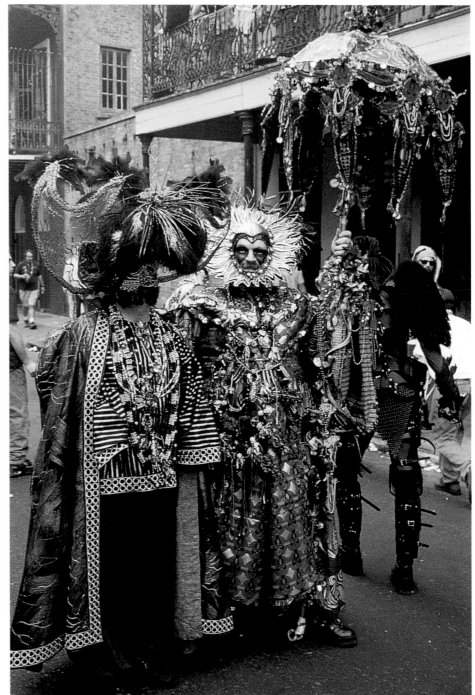

Top:
Masks for Sale
Mardi Gras
New Orleans, Louisiana
1999
Photo: Jim Pieper

Above & right:
Masked Participants
Mardi Gras
New Orleans, Louisiana
1999
Photo: Jim Pieper

MEXICO

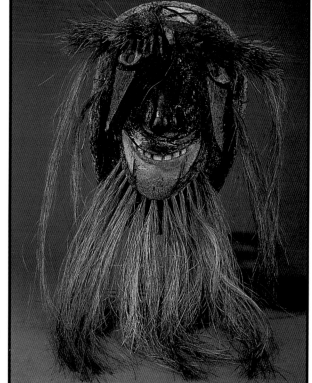

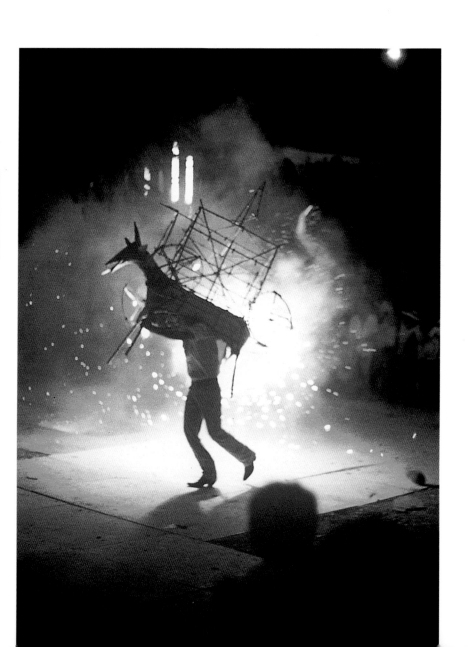

Right:
Pascola Mask
Dance of the Pascola or
"old men of the fiesta"
(Jacobsen, CF, p. 19).
Polychrome wood and
hair, 7.25 inches.
Mayo People
Potam, Sonora, Mexico
Ca. mid 20th century
Private collection

Far right:
Dance Bull
Fireworks explode from
a bull dancer, in a church
yard.
Mexico
1980s
Photo: Jim Pieper

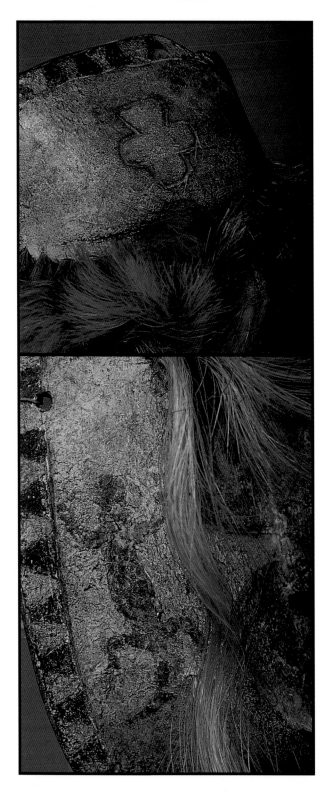

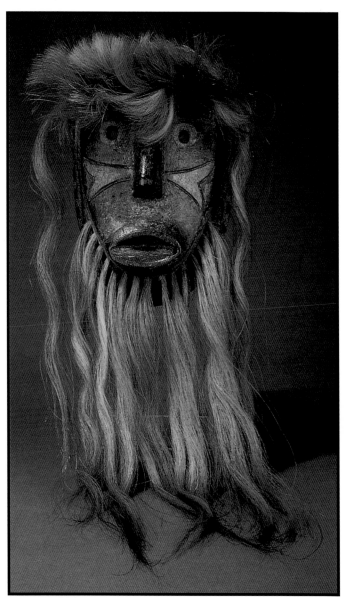

The first objects we collected related to our interest in the cultures of Latin America. As we enjoyed having these indigenous objects (masks, Santos, ceramics, textiles, etc.) in our home, we learned more about them and extended our knowledge to other societies and their unique spiritual and artistic creations. Having these artifacts in our home gives us great pleasure and continues to remind us of the many interesting and wonderful cultures in this world.

Annette and Seymour Bird

Pascola Mask
Dance of the Pascola. Polychrome wood
and hair, 7.5 inches.
Mayo People
Vicamp, Sonora, Mexico
Ca. early to mid 20th century
Private collection

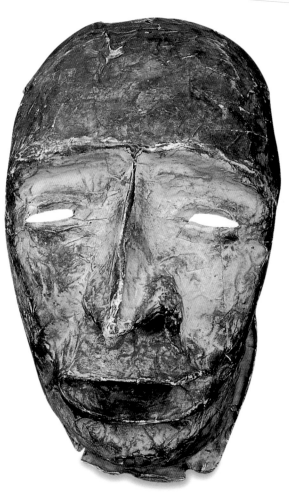

Soldier or Judas Mask
Polychrome papier-mâché mask that would have been used during Lenten ceremonies. They are normally destroyed at the conclusion of the ceremony. 8.75 inches.
Cora People
Nayarit, Mexico
Ca. late 20th century
Collection of Larry and Sandy Roseman

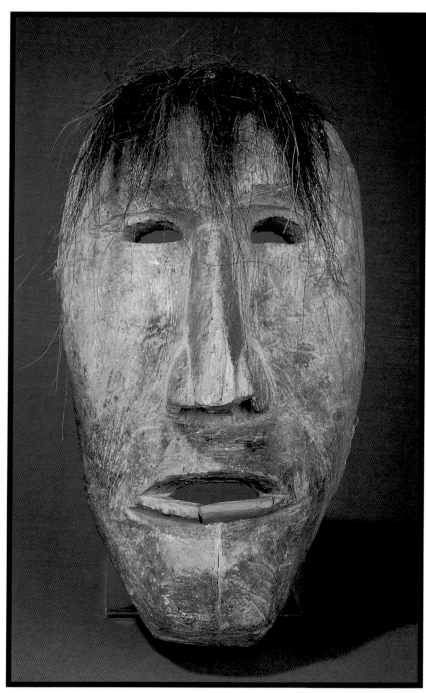

Cora Mask
Wooden masks such as this were replaced in the Cora culture in the 1950s by papier-mâché. Polychrome wood and hair, 10 inches.
Cora People
San Barsito, Nayarit, Mexico
Ca. early 20th century
Collection of Jim and Jeanne Pieper

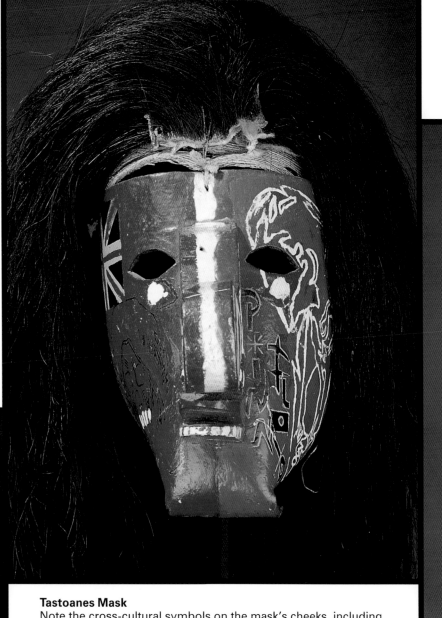

Tastoanes Mask
Note the cross-cultural symbols on the mask's cheeks, including the English Union Jack and Pink Floyd of rock 'n roll. Polychrome wood, leather, woven hat, and animal tail. 11 inches (head only).
Jalisco, Mexico
Ca. mid 20th century
Collection of Diane and Ernie Wolfe III

Right:
Viejito (Old Man) Mask
An old dance that may have pre-historic origins in ancient ritual where human skins were worn by the priests. Polychrome wood, hair, and foil, 6.5 inches.
Michoacan, Mexico
Ca. early to mid 20th century
Collection of Jim and Jeanne Pieper

Below:
Devil Mask
Human hair tops the mask, which was used in many ceremonies, including the Pastorelas. Polychrome wood, horn, canvas, hair, and leather, 8 inches.
Michoacan, Mexico
Ca. 18th to 19th century
Collection of Jim and Jeanne Pieper

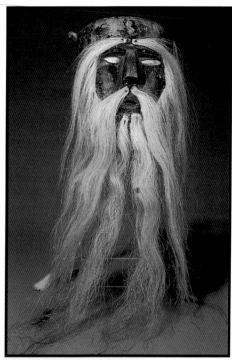

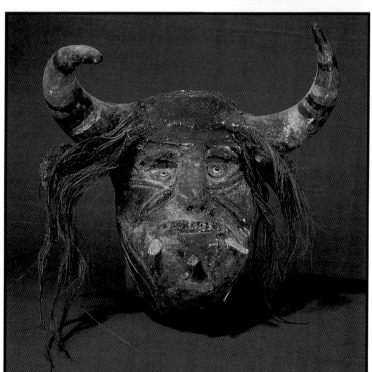

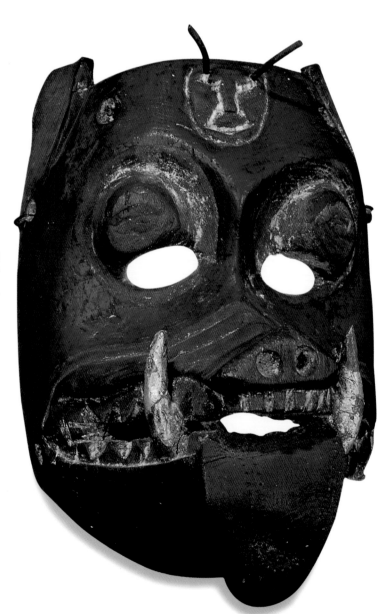

Pig Devil Mask
Notice that on the pig's forehead is a small Devil. This would allow a mask to be danced as an old pre-Christian spirit, while placating the observing Catholic priests that the mask represented the devil. Used in many ceremonies, including Pastorelas. Polychromed wood, leather, nails, and metal, 8.5 inches.
Michoacan, Mexico
Ca. early to mid 20th century
Collection of Jim and Jeanne Pieper

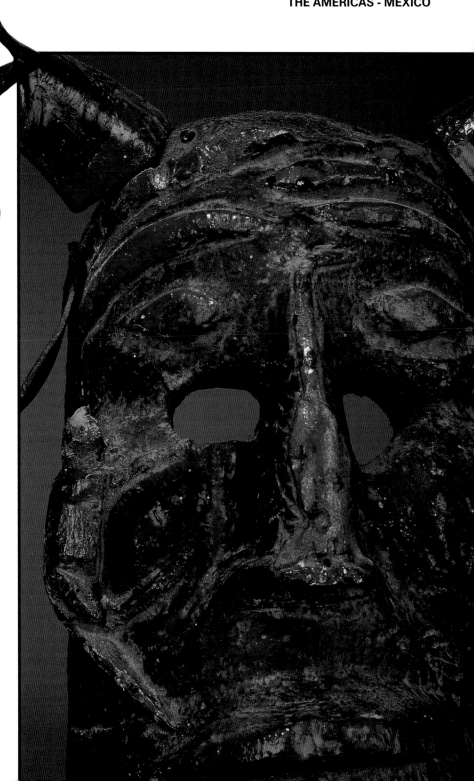

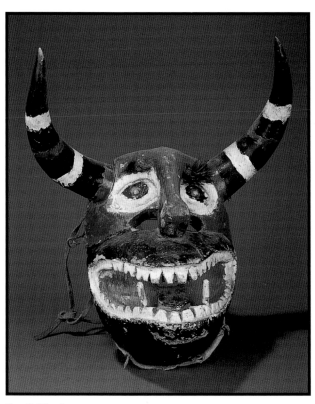

Devil Mask
Various ceremonies and in the Pastorelas. Polychrome wood, horn, leather, and nails, 13.75 inches.
Maravatio, Michoacan, Mexico
Ca. mid 20th century
Collection of Jim and Jeanne Pieper

Devil Mask
Participates in various ceremonies, dances, and the Pastorelas. Polychromed wood, horn, and animal fur, with marbles for irises, 9.25 inches.
San Felipe, Guanajuato, Mexico
Ca. mid 20th century
Collection of Jim and Jeanne Pieper

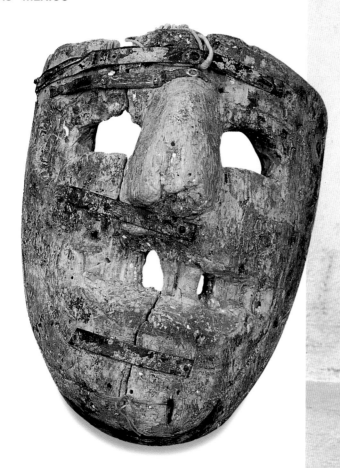

Above:
Tlacololero (Plantation Boss) Mask
Dance of Tlacololero, his dance step based on putting seed into the ground.
Polychromed wood, metal, and string, 9 inches.
State of Mexico, Mexico
Ca. early 20th century
Collection of Jim and Jeanne Pieper

Right:
Tlacololero (Plantation Boss) Mask
During the dance, the Tlacololeros frequently use whips on each other. Often you will find the masks battered and frayed.
Mexico
1980s
Photo: Jim Pieper

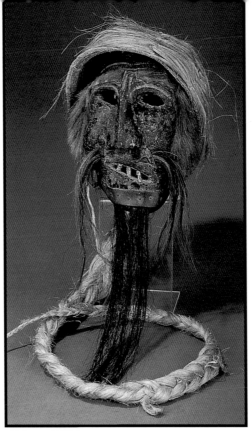

Shepherd Mask
One of the shepherds who is present for the birth of Jesus in the Dance of the Pastorelas. Polychrome wood, fur, hair, fiber, and leather, 9 inches (head only).
State of Mexico, Mexico
Ca. early 20th century
Collection of Jim and Jeanne Pieper

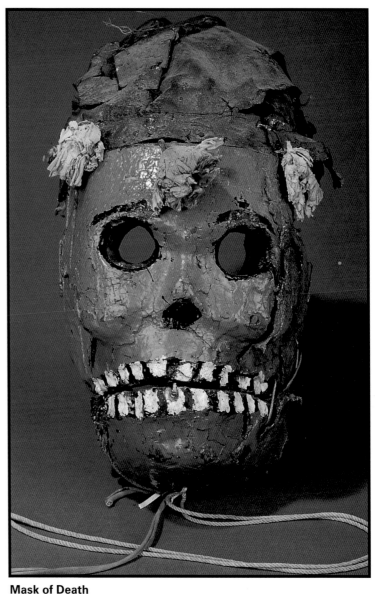

Mask of Death
Used in many different ceremonies. Wood, leather, soccer ball, paper, thread, twine, and nails. The mask features a movable jaw with part of old soccer ball for cap. Extensive repairs.
State of Mexico, Mexico
Ca. late 19th to early 20th century
Collection of Jim and Jeanne Pieper

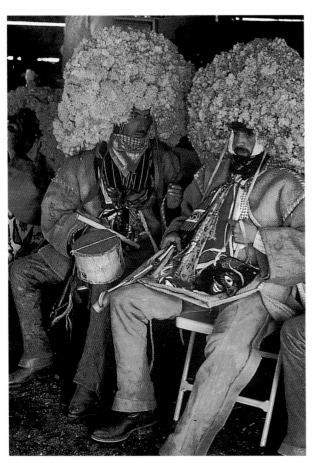

Tlacololeros at Rest
Two Tlacololeros rest in the their leather costumes with their heads covered with golden marigolds.
Guerrero, Mexico
1980s
Photo: Jim Pieper

Chinelo Mask
Danza de Chinelos (those who move their hips) *(Jacobsen, CF, p. 16)*. Painted mesh face, applied fiber for the beard and eyebrows, woven straw hat covered with velvet, with beads and sequined and beaded applique, and fringe. 20.25 inches.
Tepoztlan, Morelos, Mexico
Ca. late 1970s
Collection of Tom and Alma Pirazzini

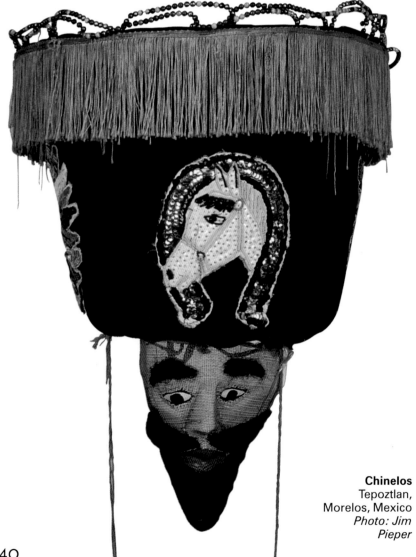

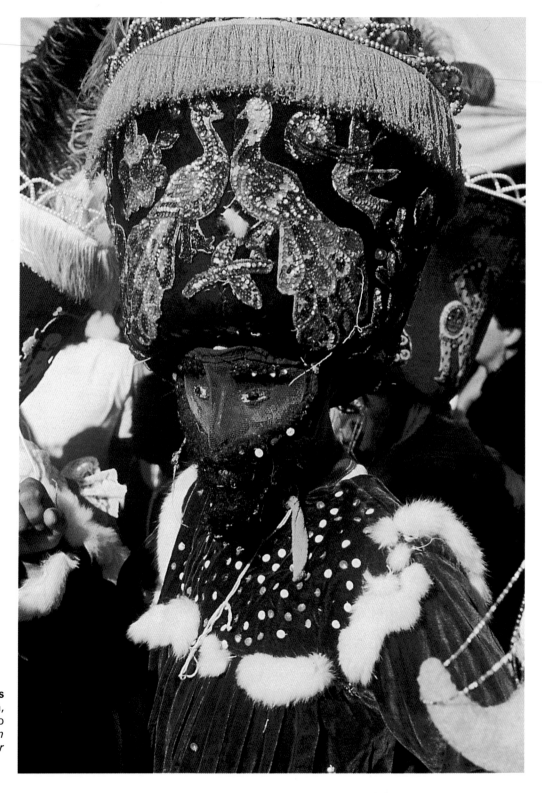

Chinelos
Tepoztlan,
Morelos, Mexico
*Photo: Jim
Pieper*

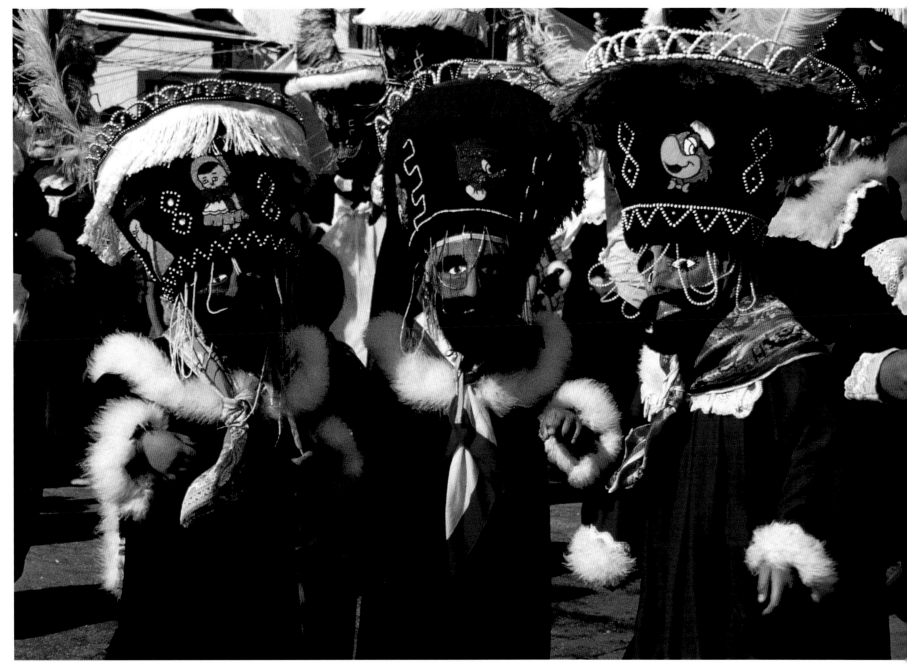

Chinelos
Three dancers wearing Chinelos masks.
Tepoztlan, Morelos, Mexico
Photo: Jim Pieper

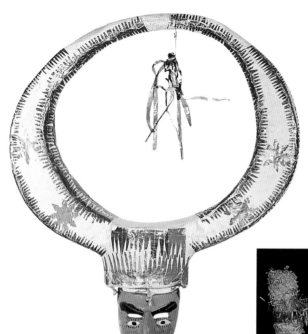

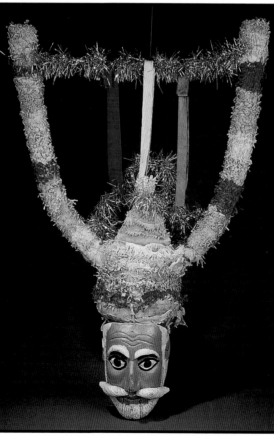

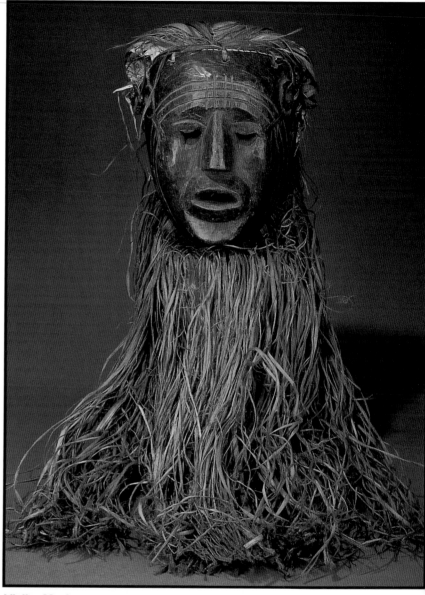

Above:
Pilato (Pontius Pilate) Mask
Dance of the Moors and Christians.
Polychrome wood mask, papier-mâché
headpiece with foil and cellophane, 30
inches.
Totoltepec, Guerrero, Mexico
Ca. mid to late 20th century
Collection of Tom and Alma Pirazzini

Right:
Saborio Dance Character Mask
Dance of the Moors and Christians.
Polychrome wood, willow and twine
frame covered with cloth and paper,
aluminum garland, ribbon, and bells.
38.5 inches.
Nahuas People
Zompahuacan, Guerrero, Mexico
Ca. mid to late 20th century
Collection of Tom and Alma Pirazzini

Viejito Mask
Old man mask that shows strong stylization,
influenced by the African slaves who were
brought to Mexico. Polychrome wood and
fiber, 7 inches (head only).
Ca. late 19th to early 20th century
Tabasco, Mexico
Collection of Jim and Jeanne Pieper

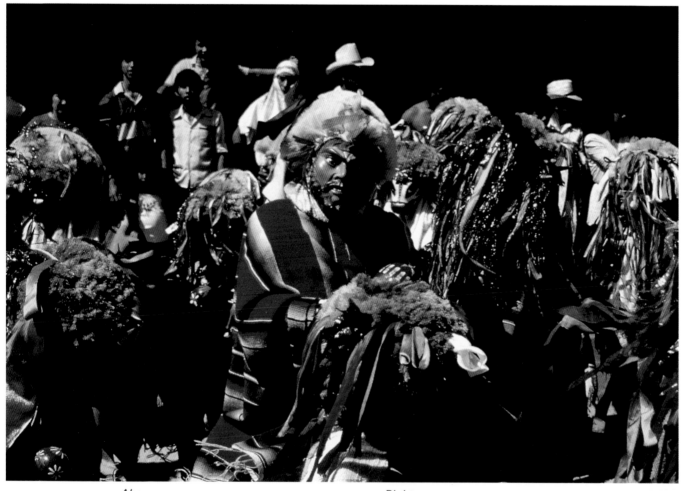

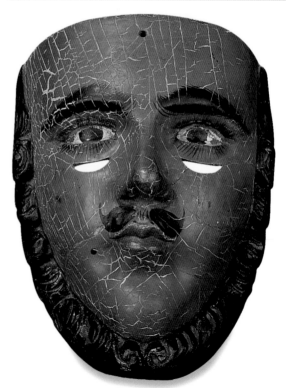

I collect because I am compelled to...it's an obsession, really. My major interest is in tribal art. I collect primarily for the pure aesthetic enjoyment of the object. However I suspect there is, in part, a more primal reason. Tribal art objects are often imbued with great spiritual power by their makers or owners.

Will Hughes

Above:
Parachico Dance
Patron Parachico dancer dances with bulls.
Suchiapa, Chiapas, Mexico
1980s
Photo: Jim Pieper

Right:
Parachico Mask
Parachico means "for the boy." The festival is based on the legend of Doria Maria de Angelo thanking Saint Sebastian for curing her sick son. Polychromed wood and eye lashes, 8 inches.
Zoque People
Chiapa De Corso, Chiapas, Mexico
Ca. mid 20th century
Collection of Jim and Jeanne Pieper

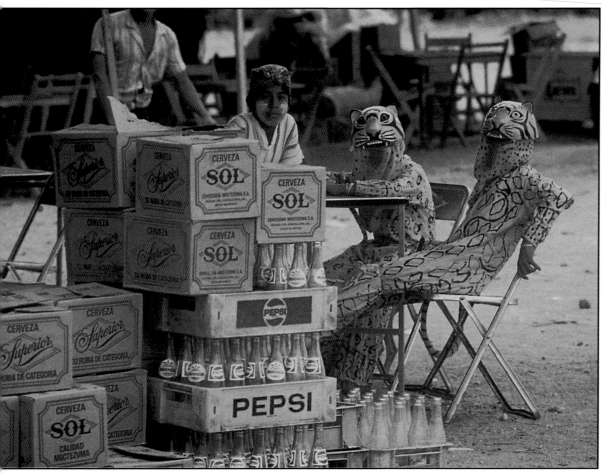

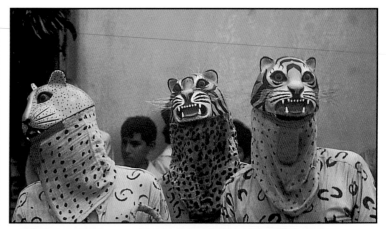

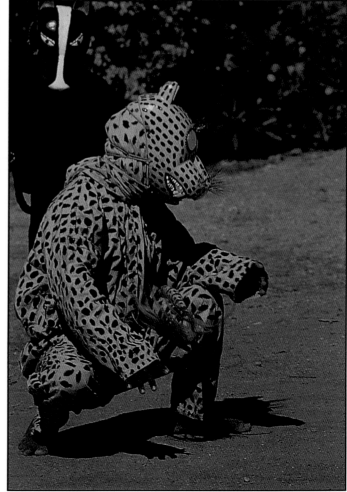

Above:
Have a Beer
Two tigers relax. Even though tigers are not indigenous to Mexico, television and magazines in our modern world have merged the tiger of India, the lion of Africa, and the Jaguar of Mexico into the same dance participant. The tiger is a part of other dances including the Dance of the Giant (Christian) and the Dance of the Deer (indigenous).
Suchiapa, Chiapas, Mexico
1980s
Photo: Jim Pieper

Above right:
Tigers
Suchiapa, Chiapas, Mexico
1980s
Photo: Jim Pieper

Right:
Tiger and Dog
Both members of an ancient hunt drama that is acted out in many forms throughout Mexico. In this small village above Oaxaca it is a festive hide-and-seek, with the tiger hiding on roofs and water tanks, while the hunter, the wife, and dog search for him amidst the laughter of the village.
Oaxaca, Mexico
1995
Photo: Jim Pieper

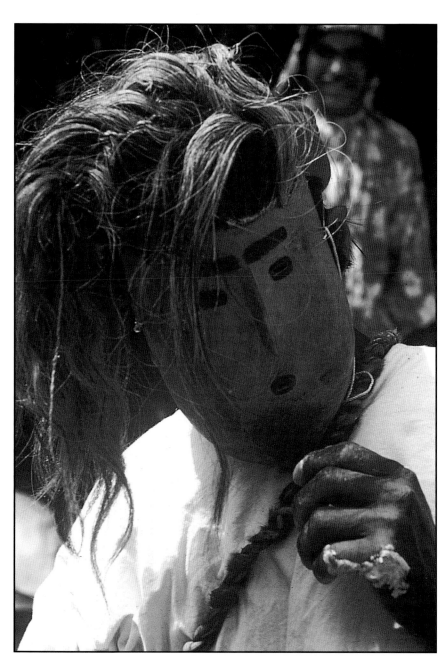

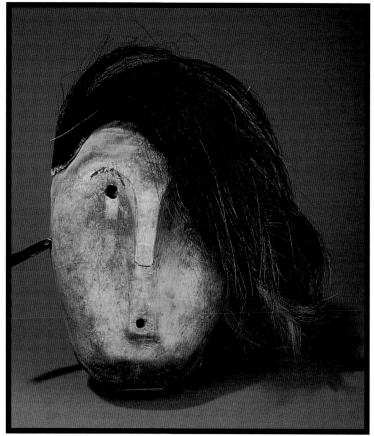

Above:

Tarahumara Mask
Polychrome wood and hair, 9.25 inches.
Tarahumara People
Mexico
Ca. mid to early 20th century
Photo Jim Pieper

Left:

Tarahumara
The Tarahumara people are the last of the cave
dwelling cultures in the Western Hemisphere.
Tarahumara People
Mexico
1985
Photo: Jim Pieper

GUATEMALA

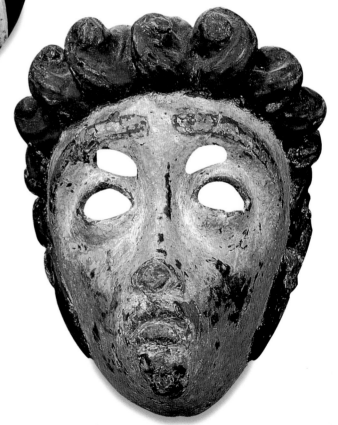

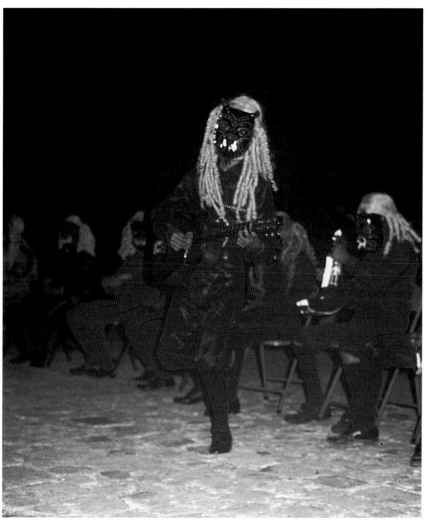

Devils
Dance of 24 Devils. The photo
portrays the devils arguing with an
angel over the soul of a Christian.
Antiqua, Guatemala
1980s
Photo: Jim Pieper

Above:
Devil Mask
Dance of 24 Devils. Poly-
chrome wood, 29.25 inches.
Guatemala
Ca. mid 20th century
*Collection of Jim and Jeanne
Pieper*

Right:
Monkey Mask
The monkey is an element of
pre-Christian dance ritual. He
is a participant in the Deer
and 24 Devil dances among
others. Polychrome wood,
7.5 inches.
Alta Vera Paz, Guatemala
Ca. 18th to 19th century
*Collection of Jim and Jeanne
Pieper*

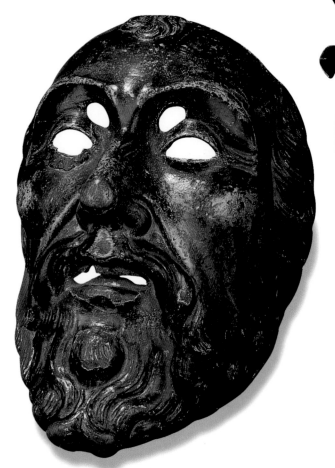

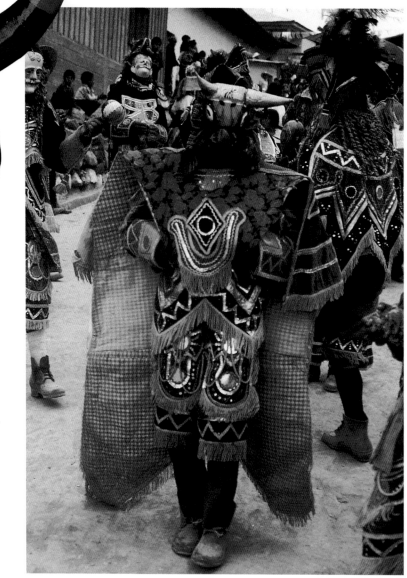

Moor Mask
Dance of the Moors and Christians.
Polychrome wood, 9.5 inches.
Alta Vera Paz, Guatemala
Ca. 18th to 19th century
Collection of Jim and Jeanne Pieper

Above:
Torito (Bull) Mask
Dance of the Torito includes
Spanish soldiers and frequently
Alvarado as participants. The bull
may also be present in the Dance
of the Mexicano. Polychrome
wood with glass eyes, 7.75 inches.
Central Highlands, Guatemala
Ca. mid 20th century
*Collection of Jim and Jeanne
Pieper*

Right:
Torito
Dance of the Torito
Guatemala
1980s
Photo: Jim Pieper

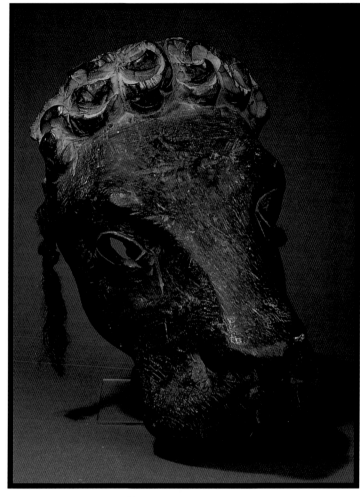

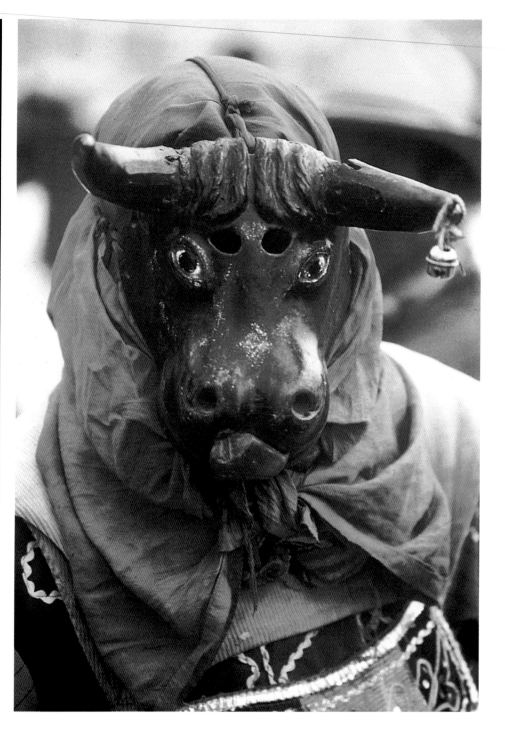

Above:
Lion or Bull Mask
Deer Dance or Dance of the Torito. Wood,
10.5 inches.
Quiche, Guatemala
Ca. late 19th to early 20th century
Collection of Jim and Jeanne Pieper

Right:
Dance of the Torito
A bull's head with brightly colored ribbons.
Guatemala
1980
Photo: Jim Pieper

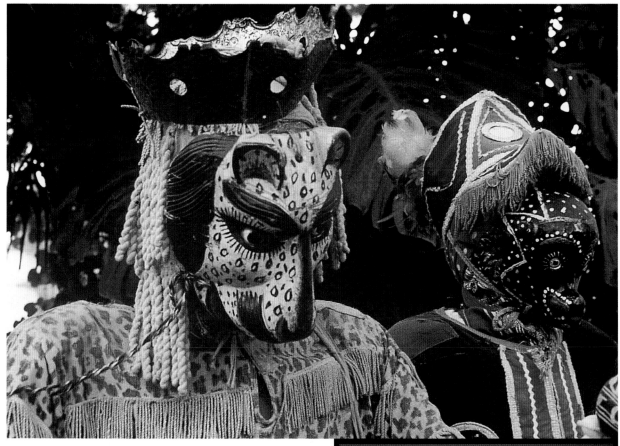

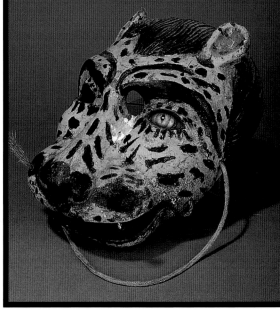

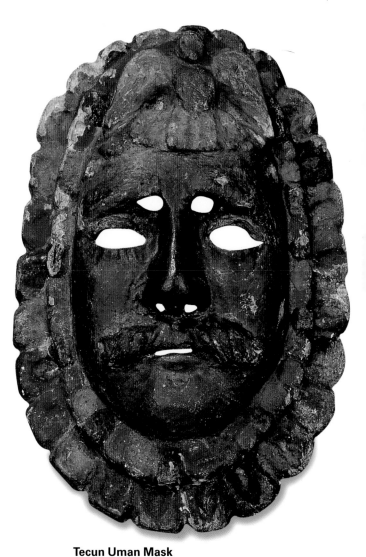

Above:
Tiger and Monkey
Dance of the Deet
Guatemala City, Guatemala
1970s
Photo: Jim Pieper

Right:
Tiger Mask
Deer Dance. Polychrome wood and
glass, with a movable jaw and dog
teeth, 8 inches.
Totonicapan, Guatemala
Ca. early 20th century
Collection of Jim and Jeanne Pieper

Tecun Uman Mask
Indigenous chief in the Dance of the
Conquest where he will fight Alvarado.
Polychrome wood, 9.5 inches.
Totonicapan, Guatemala
Ca. early 20th century
Collection of Jim and Jeanne Pieper

149

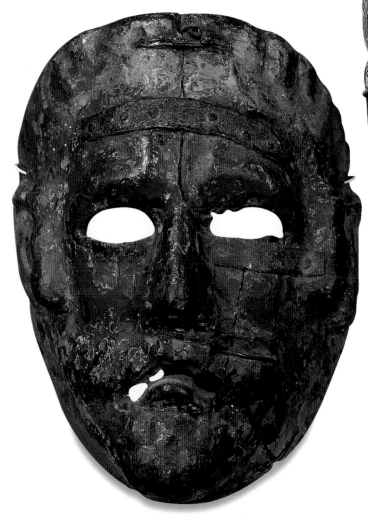

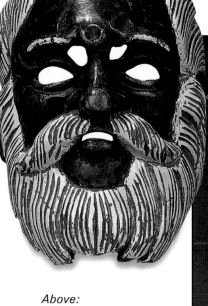

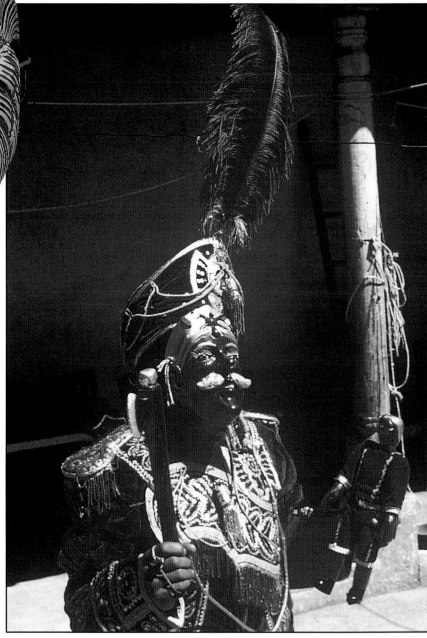

Above:
Patron Mask
The leader in many dances including Torito and Mexicano. Poly-chrome wood, 7.0 inches. Totonicapan, Guatemala Ca. mid to late 19th century
Collection of Jim and Jeanne Pieper

Right:
Ajitz or Shaman
Dance of the Conquest Totonicapan, Guatemala 1980s
Photo: Jim Pieper

Ajitz or Brujo Mask
A pre-historic shaman or healer who appears in the Dance of the Conquest. Mask shows the wear and repair from over 50 to 75 years of use. Polychrome wood, wire, and metal, 6 inches.
Totonicapan, Guatemala
Ca. mid 19th century
Collection of Jim and Jeanne Pieper

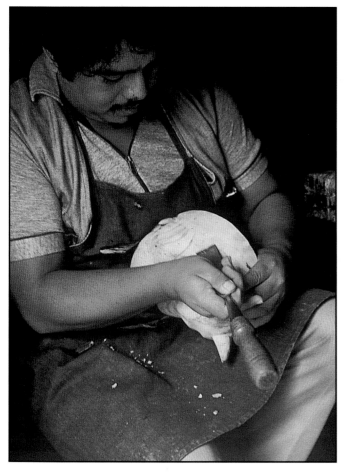

Francisco Son Garcia, a third generation carver. It takes about eight days to carve the average mask.
San Cristobal Totonicapan, Guatemala
1980s
Photo: Jim Pieper

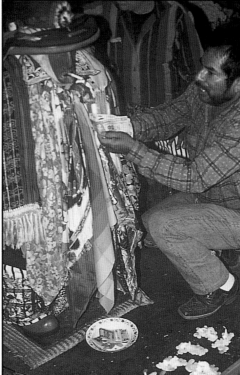

Maximon/San Simeon
The life-size Mayan/Christian deity receives ceremonial offerings.
Mayan People
Santiago Atitlan, Guatemala
1990s
Photo: Jim Pieper

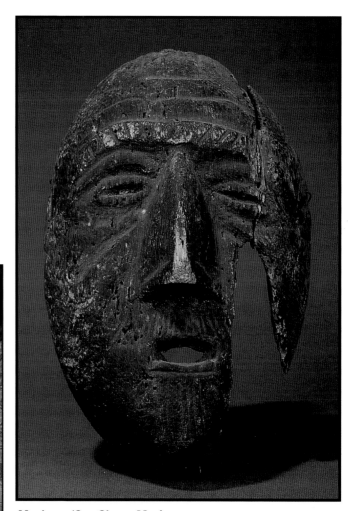

Maximon/San Simon Mask
This mask is used on a life size figure who, when prayed to in the indigenous dialect, is called Maximon and represents Mayan Deities. When prayed to in Spanish, he is then referred to as San Simon and represents a pantheon of Catholic Saints. He is ceremonially hung as Judas during Lent. Wood, 8 inches.
Santiago Atitlan, Guatemala
Ca. early 20th century
Collection of Jim and Jeanne Pieper

HONDURAS

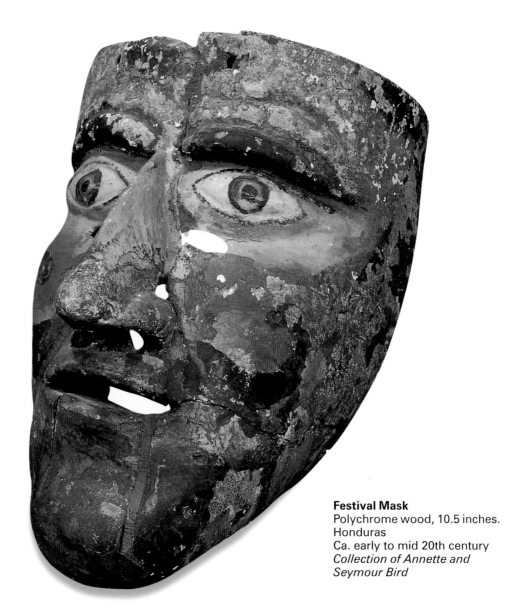

I have been a collector most of my life. Stamp collecting ignited my interest of world cultures. During my first travels to Mexico in the early '60s, I became enamoured with the art, especially pre-Columbian and the folk art traditions, which derive from ancient rituals.

In 1972, on a trip to Mexico, my wife and I bought our first masks. However, it wasn't until the '80s, inspired by the collections of some of the participants in this exhibit, that we became more serious about our own collecting.

Tom Pirazzini

Festival Mask
Polychrome wood, 10.5 inches.
Honduras
Ca. early to mid 20th century
*Collection of Annette and
Seymour Bird*

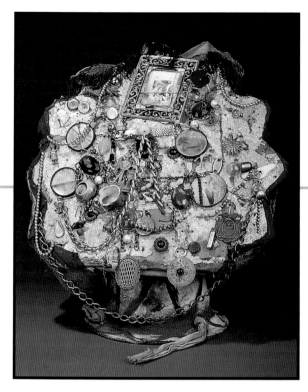

ECUADOR

Head Cover
Harvest/ Corpus Christi
Ceremony headdress.
Mixed media, 19 inches
high, 18 inches diameter.
Ecuador
Ca. mid to late 20th
century
*Collection of Jim and
Jeanne Pieper*

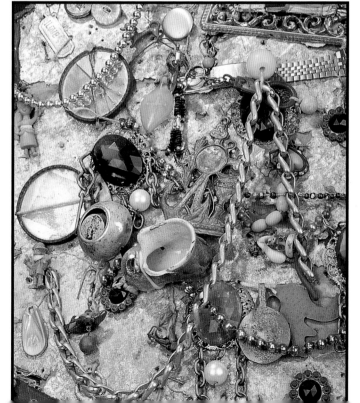

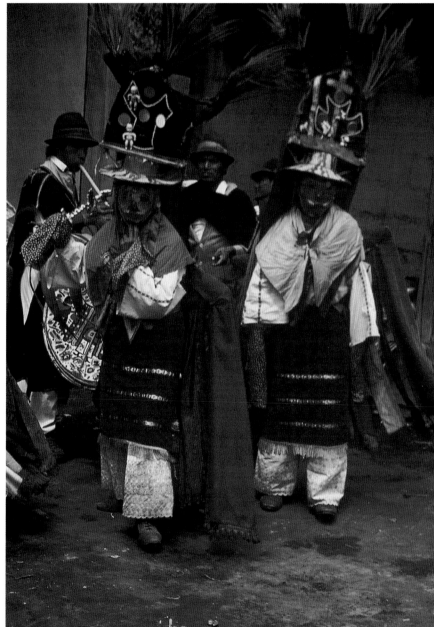

Harvest/Corpus Christi Ceremony
Tunguralura, Ecuador
1995
Photo: Jim Pieper

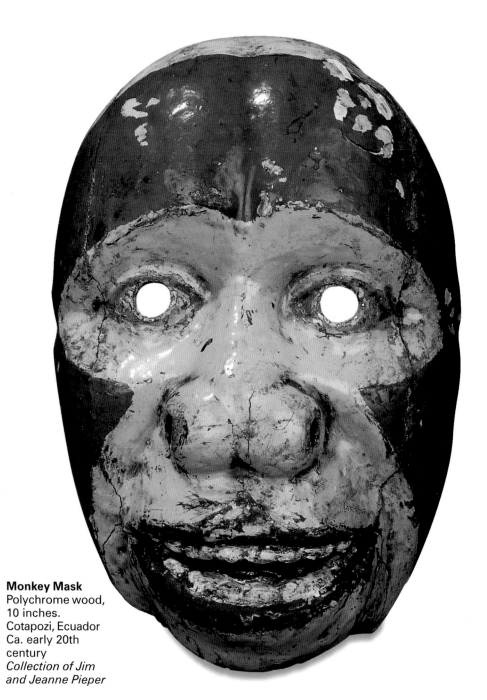

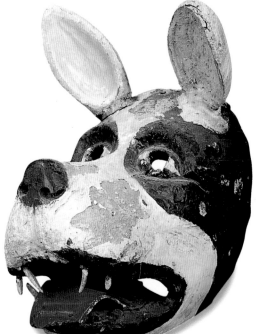

Dog Mask
Dance of the Hunt.
Polychrome wood
and leather, 11 inches
deep, 9 inches wide.
Cotapozi, Ecuador
Ca. early 20th century
*Collection of Jim and
Jeanne Pieper*

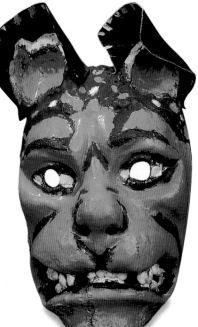

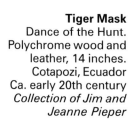

Tiger Mask
Dance of the Hunt.
Polychrome wood and
leather, 14 inches.
Cotapozi, Ecuador
Ca. early 20th century
*Collection of Jim and
Jeanne Pieper*

Monkey Mask
Polychrome wood,
10 inches.
Cotapozi, Ecuador
Ca. early 20th
century
*Collection of Jim
and Jeanne Pieper*

Diablo Umo
The ornate mask is danced by Senorita
Valdiorior, the daughter of a man running for
the Ecuadorian House of Representatives.
Tabacundo, Ecuador
1995
Photo: Jim Pieper

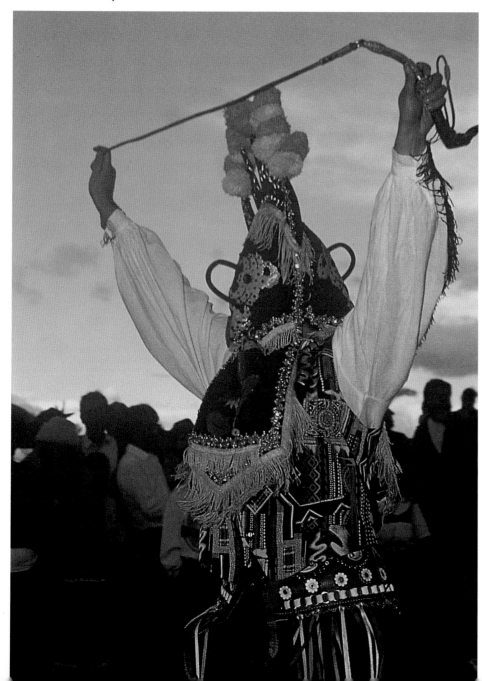

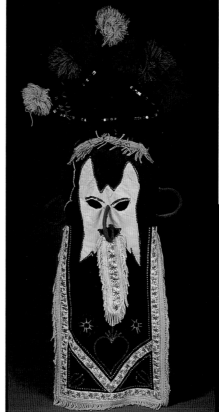

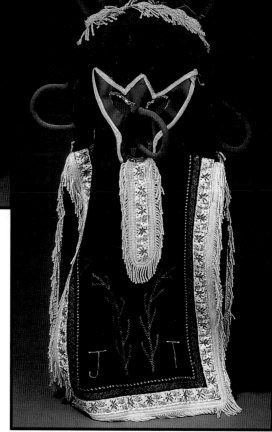

Diablo Umo Mask
Fabric, yarn, and fringe,
40.5 inches.
Tabacundo, Ecuador
Ca. late 20th century
*Collection of Jim and
Jeanne Pieper*

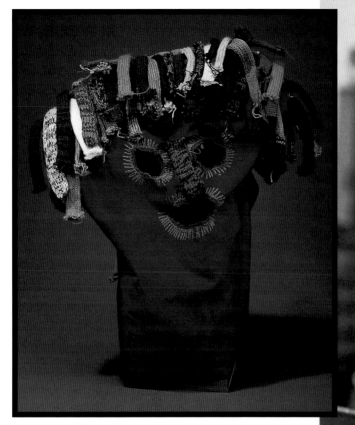

Above:
Diablo Umo Mask
Represents Sun deity with Christian overlay of devil. This simple mask form is used by the indigenous people and is danced for Christmas, and for Saints Peter's, Paul's and John's Days. Fabric and yarn, 16.5 inches.
Tabacundo, Ecuador
Ca. late 20th century
Collection of Jim and Jeanne Pieper

Right:
Diablo Umo
Dancer offers a drink to the photographer.
1995
Tabacundo, Ecuador
Photo: Jim Pieper

BOLIVIA

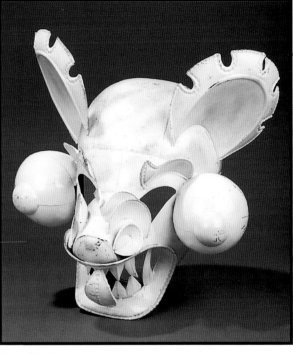

Bear Mask
Dance of Diablado. Tin, 12.5 inches deep, 13.25 inches wide.
Bolivia
Ca. late 20th century
Collection of Hope and Roy Turney

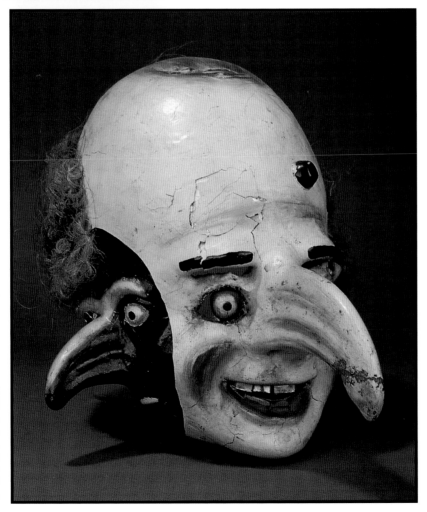

Three-Faced Mask
Faces on both cheeks used in the Dance of Diablado. Composition, fiber, hair, mirrors, 12.5 inches.
Bolivia
Ca. mid 20th century
Collection of Ann and Monroe Morgan

Fish Head Helmet
One of the animals in the
Dance of Diablado. Recycled
tin, 14.75 inches.
Bolivia
Ca. 20th century
*Collection Ann and Monroe
Morgan*

Devil Mask
The most important mask of the Dance
of Diablado to honor the Virgin of the
Mineshaft (Virgen del Selaven).
Recycled tin alcohol cans, 19 inches
deep, 16.5 inches wide.
Bolivia
Ca. late 20th century
Collection of Hope and Roy Turney

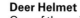

Deer Helmet
One of the animal characters
in the Dance of Diablado.
Composition with fabric
covering, 13 inches diameter,
14.5 inches wide.
Bolivia
Ca. mid 20th century
*Collection Ann and Monroe
Morgan*

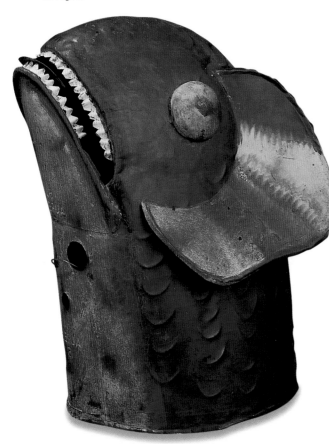

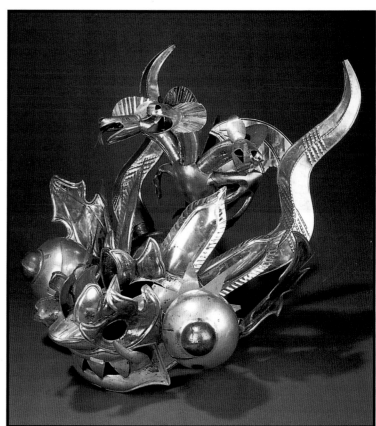

Right:
Diablo Mask
This mask is used in the Dance of Diablado.
Composition, tin, plaster, plastic baseballs for eyes,
leather ears, and paint, 18 inches high.
Bolivia
Ca. mid 20th century
Collection Ann and Monroe Morgan

Below:
Supay Mask
Believed by the tin miners to be an underground
spirit who is not all evil or all good. In some
contexts he is also considered to be Jesus. It is said
that he can reveal treasures or cause mine disas-
ters. Recycled tin. 16.5 inches wide.
Oruro, Bolivia
Ca. late 20th century
Collection of Hope and Roy Turney

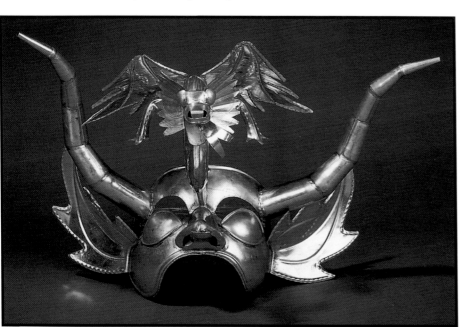

*We collect because we enjoy the challenge and
adventure of the hunt (i.e., of searching for and finding things); we like to learn about diverse cultures
by traveling to see them and by learning about the
items they make; we like to have beautiful, interesting, human culture art work in our home; we want
to preserve the dying ethnic arts for posterity and
for other to see and appreciate.*
Private Collectors

BIBLIOGRAPHY

Brabson, Oscar T. *Hopi Indian Kachina Dolls.* Tucson: Treasure Chest Publictions, 1992.

Bruggmann, Maximilien, and Peter R. Gerber. *Indians of the Northwest Coast.* New York: Facts on File, 1987.

Bushell, Raymond. *Netsuke Masks.* New York: Weatherhill, 1985

Cole, Aniakor. *Igbo Arts: Community and Cosmos.* Los Angeles: Museum of Cultural History, University of California at Los Angeles, 1984.

Colton, Harold S. *Hopi Kachina Dolls with a Key to their Identification.* Albuquerque: University of New Mexico Press, 1959.

D'Alleva, Anne. *Arts of the Pacific Islands.* New York: Harry Abrams, 1998.

Dockstader, Frederick J. *The Kachina and the White Man: The Influences of White Culture on the Hopi Kachina Cult.* Albuquerque: University of New Mexico Press, 1985.

_____. *Indian Art in North America.* New York: New York Graphic Society, 1961.

Fagg, William. *Nigerian Images: The Splendor of African Sculpture.* New York: Frederick A. Praeger, 1963.

Glassie, Henry. *The Spirit of Folk Art: The Girard Collection at the Museum of International Folk Art.* New York: Harry Abrams, 1995.

Goonatilleka, M.H. *Masks and Mask Systems of Sri Lanka.* Colombo: Tamarind Books, 1978.

Herold, Erich. *Tribal Masks.* London: Paul Hamlyn, 1967.

Hopfner, Gerd. *Masken aus Ceylon.* Berlin: Museum fur Volkerkinde, 1969.

Huet, Michel. *The Dances of Africa.* New York: Harry C. Abrams, Inc., 1996.

Jacobson, Lori, and Donald E. Fritz. *Changing Faces: Mexican Masks in Transition.* McAllen, Texas: McAllen International Museum, 1985.

Jonaitis, Aldona. *From the Land of the Totem Poles: The Northwest Coast Indian Art Collection of the American Museum of Natural History.* New York: American Museum of Natural History, 1988.

_____, Editor. *Chiefly Feasts: The Enduring Kwakiutl Potlatch.* Seattle: University of Washington Press, 1991.

Lechuga, Ruth Deutsch. *Mascaras Tradicionales De Mexico.* Mexico: Banco Nacional de Obras y Servicios Publicos,S.N.C., 1991.

Lechuga, Ruth D., and Chloe Sayer. *Mask Art of Mexico.* San Francisco: Chronicle Books, 1994.

Lenzinger, Elsy. *The Art of Black Africa.* Greenwich, CT: New York Graphic Society, Ltd., 1972

Linton, Ralph, and Paul S. Wingert in collaboration with Rene D'Harnoncourt. *Arts of the South Seas.* New York: The Museum of Modern Art, 1946.

Mack, John. *Masks and the Art of Expression.* New York: Harry Abrams, 1994.

Maksic, Sava and Paul Meskil. *Primitive Art of New Guinea: Sepik River Basin.* Worcester, MA: Davis Publications, Inc., 1973

Markman, Roberta H. and Peter T. *Masks of the Spirit.* Los Angeles: University of California Press, 1989.

Mauldin, Barbara. *Masks of Mexico.* Sante Fe: Museum of New Mexico Press, 1999.

McFarren, Peter. *Masks of the Bolivian Andes.* La Paz, Bolivia: Banco Mercantil S.A.

Meauze, Pierre. *African Art.* Cleveland: The World Publishing Company, 1968.

Pace Gallery. *African Accumulative Sculpture.* New York: Pace Gallery, 1974.

Pauline, Denise. *African Sculpture.* New York: Viking Press, 1962.

Pieper, Jim and Jeanne. *Guatemalan Masks: The Pieper Collection.* Los Angeles: Craft and Folk Art Museum, 1988.

Robbins, Waren M. and Nancy Ingram Nooter,. *African Art in the American Collection.* Washington: The Smithsonian Institute, 1989.

Ross, Doran H. "Carnival Masquerades in Guinea-Bissau," *African Arts* Vol xxvi, Number 3, July, 1993. Los Angeles: UCLA, 1993.

Seattle Art Museum. *The Spirit Within: Northwest Coast Native Art from the John H. Hauberg Collection.* New York: Rizzoli, 1995.

Segy, Ladislas. *African Sculpture Speaks, 4th Edition.* New York: Da Capo Press, 1975.

_____. *African Sculpture.* New York: Dover Publications, 1958.

_____. *Masks of Black Africa.* New York: Dover Publications, 1976.

Sieber, Roy, and Roslyn Adele Walker. *African Art in the Cycle of Life.* Washington: The Smithsonian Institution Press, 1989.

Song, Sok-ha. *Minsok sajin ukpyolchan torots (Korean Masks).* 1975

Taylor, Meg, and Chris Rainier. *Where Masks Still Dance: New Guinea.* Boston: Little, Brown, and Company, 1996.

Underwood, Leon. *Masks of West Africa.* London: Alec Tiranti, 1964.

Wardell, Alan. *The Art of the Sepik River.* Chicago: The Art Institute of Chicago, 1971

Willett, Frank. *African Art.* New York: Thames and Hudson, 1985.

Wright, Barton. *Hopi Kachinas: The Complete Guide to Collecting Kachina Dolls.* Flagstaff: Northland Press, 1977.